Surgery at a Glance

Surgery at a Glance

PIERCE A. GRACE

MCh, FRCSI, FRCS
Professor of Surgical Science
University of Limerick
Midwestern Regional Hospital
Limerick

NEIL R. BORLEY

FRCS, FRCS (Ed)
Consultant Colorectal Surgeon
Cheltenham General Hospital
Gloucestershire

SECOND EDITION

Blackwell
Science

© 1999, 2002 by Blackwell Science Ltd
a Blackwell Publishing Company
Editorial Offices:
Osney Mead, Oxford OX2 0EL, UK
    Tel: +44 (0)1865 206206
Blackwell Science, Inc., 350 Main Street, Malden, MA 02148-5018, USA
    Tel: +1 781 388 8250
Blackwell Science Asia Pty, 54 University Street, Carlton, Victoria 3053, Australia
    Tel: +61 (0)3 9347 0300
Blackwell Wissenschafts Verlag, Kurfürstendamm 57, 10707 Berlin, Germany
    Tel: +49 (0)30 32 79 060

First published 1999
Second edition 2002
Reprinted 2003

Library of Congress Cataloging-in-Publication Data

Grace, P. A. (Pierce A.)
        Surgery at a glance / Pierce A. Grace, Neil R. Borley.—2nd ed.
            p.,   cm.—(At a glance series)
        Includes index.
        ISBN 0-632-05988-5 (pbk.)
        1. Diagnosis, Surgical—Handbooks, manuals, etc.
    2. Operations, Surgical—Handbooks, manuals, etc.
    3. Surgery—Handbooks, manuals, etc.
    I. Borley, Neil R.   II. Title.   III. Series.
        [DNLM: 1. Surgical Procedures, Operative—Handbooks.
    2. Diagnosis—Handbooks.
    WO 39 G729c 2002]
    RD35 G68 2002
    617′.9—dc21   2001052912

ISBN 0-632-05988-5

A catalogue record for this title is available from the British Library

Set in 9½/12 Times by Graphicraft Limited, Hong Kong
Printed and bound in Great Britain by MPG Books Ltd, Bodmin, Cornwall

For further information on Blackwell Science, visit our website:
www.blackwell-science.com

Contents

Preface 7

List of abbreviations 8

Part 1 Clinical presentations at a glance

1 Neck lump 10

2 Dysphagia 12

3 Haemoptysis 14

4 Breast lump 16

5 Breast pain 18

6 Nipple discharge 20

7 Haematemesis 22

8 Dyspepsia 24

9 Vomiting 26

10 Acute abdominal pain 28

11 Chronic abdominal pain 30

12 Abdominal swellings (general) 32

13 Abdominal swellings (localized): upper abdominal 34

14 Abdominal swellings (localized): lower abdominal 38

15 Jaundice 40

16 Rectal bleeding 42

17 Diarrhoea 44

18 Altered bowel habit/constipation 46

19 Groin swellings 48

20 Claudication 50

21 Acute warm painful leg 52

22 Acute 'cold' leg 54

23 Leg ulceration 56

24 Dysuria 58

25 Urinary retention 60

26 Haematuria 62

27 Scrotal swellings 64

Part 2 Surgical diseases at a glance

28 Hypoxia 66

29 Shock 68

30 SIRS 70

31 Acute renal failure 72

32 Fractures 74

33 Burns 76

34 Major trauma—basic principles 78

35 Head injury 80

36 Gastro-oesophageal reflux 84

37 Oesophageal carcinoma 86

38 Peptic ulceration 88

39 Gastric carcinoma 90

40 Malabsorption 92

41 Crohn's disease 94

42 Acute appendicitis 96

43 Diverticular disease 98

44 Ulcerative colitis 100

45 Colorectal carcinoma 102

46 Benign anal and perianal disorders 104

47 Intestinal obstruction 106

48 Abdominal hernias 108

49 Gallstone disease 110

50 Pancreatitis 114

51 Pancreatic tumours 116

52 Benign breast disease 118

53 Breast cancer 120

54 Goitre 122

55 Thyroid malignancies 124

56 Parathyroid disease 126

57 Pituitary disorders 128

58 Adrenal disorders 130

59 Skin cancer 132

60 Ischaemic heart disease 134

61 Valvular heart disease 136

62 Peripheral occlusive vascular disease 138

63 The diabetic foot 140

64 Aneurysms 142

65 Extracranial arterial disease 144

66 Deep venous thrombosis 146

67 Varicose veins 148

68 Pulmonary collapse and postoperative pneumonia 150

69 Bronchial carcinoma 152

70 Urinary tract infection 154

71 Benign prostatic hypertrophy 156

72 Renal calculi 158

73 Renal cell carcinoma 160

74 Carcinoma of the bladder 162

75 Carcinoma of the prostate 164

76 Testicular cancer 166

77 Urinary incontinence 168

78 Paediatric 'general' surgery 170

Index 173

Preface

Since it was first published in 1999, *Surgery at a Glance* has become a favourite with medical students. The book was written primarily as a learning and revision aid for students studying for the final MB examination. However, others who require an overview of clinical surgery, for example, nursing students and some postgraduate surgical students, have also found *Surgery at a Glance* useful.

This new edition follows the same format as the previous edition but it has been revised extensively without significantly increasing its size. The book is presented in two parts: Part 1 (Clinical presentations at a glance) concentrates on the symptoms and signs with which patients present, while Part 2 (Surgical diseases at a Glance) is concerned with the common surgical diseases that one is likely to see in practice (or meet in an exam!). Each of the 27 chapters in Part 1 gives a breakdown of the common causes of a particular clinical presentation, for example, abdominal pain, and this section should be especially useful when preparing for a clinical examination. Part 2 comprises 51 chapters on the common diseases encountered in surgery and should be helpful when faced with questions such as 'what do you know about carcinoma of the stomach?'. Many of the illustrations have been reworked and the text has been revised for this second edition. A new feature is the addition of Key Points and Key Investigations or Essential Management boxes to each chapter; these provide the core information a student should know for each topic. A number of new topics have been added (e.g. trauma, general paediatric surgery) and some old ones removed or amalgamated. In keeping with the format of the *at a Glance* series, each chapter is presented across a two-page spread, illustrations on the left-hand page and text on the right. The illustrations and text compliment each other to give an overview of a topic at a glance.

We have had tremendous help from several people in putting this book together. We would like to thank the many medical students who have read the book, or parts of the book, over the last five years and given us good suggestions. Books would never appear without publishers, and we would like to thank the team at Blackwell Publishing including Andrew Robinson, Fiona Goodgame, Anita Lane and Karen Moore for their encouragement, patience and professionalism in bringing the project to fruition. We thank the illustrator especially for the excellent illustrations.

Pierce Grace
Neil Borley

List of abbreviations

AAA	abdominal aortic aneurysm		Dop	dopamine
AAT	aspartate amino transferase		DPTA	diethylenetriaminepentaacetic acid
ABI	ankle–brachial pressure index		DU	duodenal ulcer
Ach	acetylcholine		DVT	deep venous thrombosis
ACN	acute cortical necrosis		DXT	deep X-ray therapy
ACTH	adrenocorticotrophic hormone		EAS	external anal sphincter
ADH	antidiuretic hormone		EBV	Epstein–Barr virus
Adr	adrenaline		ECG	electrocardiogram
AF	atrial fibrillation		ER	oestrogen receptor
AFP	α-fetoprotein		ERCP	endoscopic retrograde cholangiopancreatographic (examination)
Ag	antigen			
Alb	albumin		ESR	erythrocyte sedimentation rate
ANCA	anti-neutrophil cytoplasmic antibody		ESWL	extracorporeal shock-wave lithotripsy
ANDI	abnormalities of the normal development and involution (of the breast)		EUA	examination under anaesthesia
			FBC	full blood count
AP	anteroposterior		FCD	fibrocystic disease
APTT	activated partial thromboplastin time		FHx	family history
ARDS	adult/acute respiratory distress syndrome		FNAC	fine-needle aspiration cytology
ARF	acute renal failure		FSH	follicle-stimulating hormone
ATN	acute tubular necrosis		5-FU	5-fluorouracil
AVM	arteriovenous malfunction		γ-GT	gamma glutamyl transpeptidase
AXR	abdominal X-ray		GA	general anaesthetic
BCC	basal cell carcinoma		GCS	Glasgow Coma Scale
BCG	bacillus Calmette–Guérin		GFR	glomerular filtration rate
BE	base excess		GH	growth hormone
BP	blood pressure		GI	gastrointestinal
BPH	benign prostatic hypertrophy		GORD	gastro-oesophageal reflux disease
C&S	culture and sensitivity		GTN	glyceryl trinitrate
CABG	coronary artery bypass surgery		GU	genito-urinary
CBD	common bile duct		Hb	haemoglobin
CCF	congestive cardiac failure		β-HCG	β-human chorionic gonadotrophin
CD	*Clostridium difficile*		Hct	haematocrit
CEA	carcinoembryonic antigen		HDU	high-dependency unit
CK	creatinine kinase		HIDA	imido-diacetic acid
CLO	*Campylobacter*-like organism		HLA	human leucocyte antigen
CMV	cytomegalovirus		Hx	history
CNS	central nervous system		IBS	irritable bowel syndrome
COCP	combined oral contraceptive pill		ICP	intracranial pressure
COPD	chronic obstructive pulmonary disease		ICS	intercostal space
CPK-MB	creatine phosphokinase (cardiac type)		ICU	intensive care unit
CRC	colorectal carcinoma		IgG	immunoglobulin G
CRF	chronic renal failure		IPPV	intermittent positive pressure ventilation
CRP	C-reactive protein		ITP	idiopathic thrombocytopaenic purpura
CSF	cerebrospinal fluid		IVC	inferior vena cava
CT	computed tomography		IVU	intravenous urogram
CVA	cerebrovascular accident		JVP	jugular venous pulse
CVP	central venous pressure		LA	local anaesthetic
CXR	chest X-ray		LAD	left anterior descending
D_2	type 2 dopaminergic receptors		LATS	long-acting thyroid stimulating (factor)
DIC	disseminated intravascular coagulation		LCA	left coronary artery
DMSA	dimercaptosuccinic acid		LDH	lactate dehydrogenase

LFT	liver function test	PTC	percutaneous transhepatic cholangiography
LH	luteinizing hormone	PTH	parathyroid hormone
LH-RH	LH-releasing hormone	PUD	peptic ulcer disease
LIF	left iliac fossa	PUO	pyrexia of unknown origin
LOC	loss of consciousness	PV	per vaginum
LOS	lower oesophageal sphincter	PVD	peripheral vascular disease
LPS	lipopolysaccharide	RBC	red blood cell
LSE	left sternal edge	RCC	renal cell carcinoma
LSF	lesser sciatica foramen	RIA	radioimmunoassay
LUQ	left upper quadrant	RIF	right iliac fossa
LV	left ventricle	RLN	recurrent laryngeal nerve
LVF	left ventricular failure	RPLND	retroperitoneal lymph node dissection
MC+S	microscopy cultures and sensitivity	RUQ	right upper quadrant
MCP	metacarpophalangeal	RV	right ventricle
MEN	multiple endocrine neoplasia	RVF	right ventricular failure
MI	myocardial infarction	Rx	treatment
MIBG	*meta*-iodo-benzyl guanidine	SCC	squamous cell carcinoma
MM	malignant melanoma	SFJ	sapheno-femoral junction
MND	motor neurone disease	SGOT	serum glutamic oxalacetic transaminase
MODS	multiple organ dysfunction syndrome	SIADH	syndrome of inappropriate antidiuretic hormone
MRCP	magnetic resonance cholangio-pancreatography	SIRS	systemic inflammatory response syndrome
MRI	magnetic resonance imaging	SLE	systemic lupus erythematosus
MS	multiple sclerosis	SLN	superior laryngeal nerve
MSH	melanocyte-stimulating hormone	STD	sodium tetradecyl
MSU	mid-stream urine	SVC	superior vena cava
MT	major trauma	Sxr	skull X-ray
MTP	metatarsophalangeal	T_3	tri-iodothyronine
MUGA	multiple uptake gated analysis	T_4	thyroxine
NAdr	noradrenaline	TB	tuberculosis
NG	nasogastric	TCC	transitional cell carcinoma
NSAID	non-steroidal anti-inflammatory drug	TED	thrombo-embolic deterrent
NSU	non-specific urethritis	TIA	transient ischaemic attack
OA	osteoarthritis	TNM	tumour, node, metastasis (staging)
OGD	oesophago-gastro-duodenoscopy	t-PA	tissue plasminogen activator
OGJ	oesophago-gastric junction	TPHA	treponema pallidum haemagglutination (test)
PA	posteroanterior	TPR	temperature, pulse, respiration
PAF	platelet activating factor	TSH	thyroid-stimulating hormone
PCA	patient-controlled analgesia	TURP	transurethral resection of the prostate
PCV	packed cell volume	TURT	transurethral resection of tumour
PE	pulmonary embolism	UC	ulcerative colitis
PHx	past history	UDT	undescended testis
PIP	proximal interphalangeal	U+E	urea and electrolytes
PL	prolactin	UTI	urinary tract infection
PMN	polymorphonuclear leucocyte	VA	visual acuity
POVD	peripheral occlusive vascular disease	VHL	von Hippel–Lindau
PPI	proton pump inhibitor	VIP	vasoactive intestinal peptide
PPL	postphlebitic limb	VMA	vanillyl mandelic acid
PR	per rectum	VSD	ventricular septal defect
PSA	prostate-specific antigen	WCC	white cell count
PT	prothrombin time		

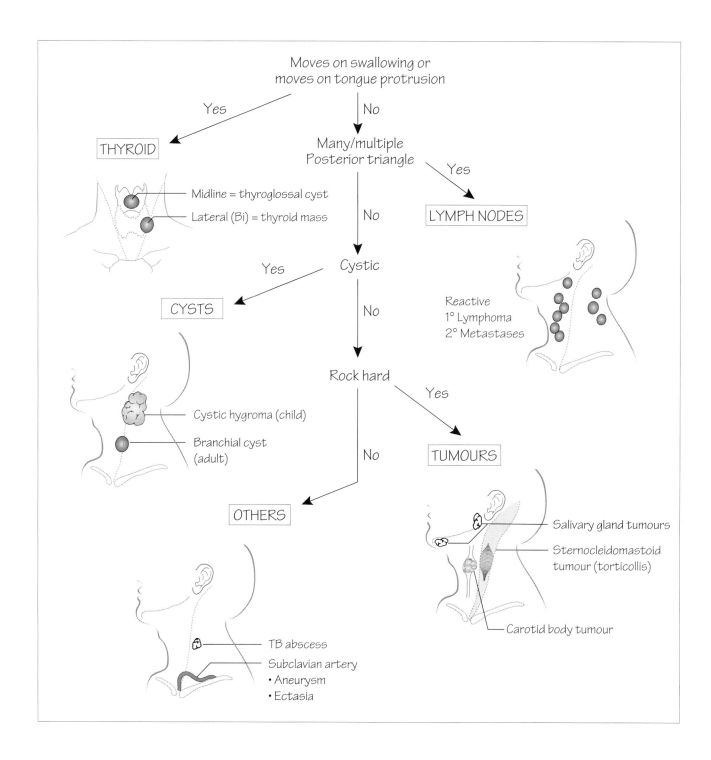

Definition

A neck lump is any congenital or acquired mass arising in the anterior or posterior triangles of the neck between the clavicles inferiorly and the mandible and base of the skull superiorly.

KEY POINTS

- Thyroid swellings move upwards (with the trachea) on swallowing.
- Most abnormalities of the neck are visible as swellings.
- Ventral lumps attached to the hyoid bone, such as thyroglossal cysts, move upwards with both swallowing and protrusion of the tongue.
- Multiple lumps are almost always lymph nodes.
- Don't forget a full head and neck examination, including the oral cavity, in all cases of lymphadenopathy.

Differential diagnosis

- 50% of neck lumps are thyroid in origin.
- 40% of neck lumps are caused by malignancy (80% metastatic usually from primary lesion above the clavicle; 20% primary neoplasms: lymphomas, salivary gland tumours).
- 10% of neck lumps are inflammatory or congenital in origin.

Thyroid
- Goitre, cyst, neoplasm.

Neoplasm
- Metastatic carcinoma.
- Primary lymphoma.
- Salivary gland tumour.
- Sternocleidomastoid tumour.
- Carotid body tumour.

Inflammatory
- Acute infective adenopathy.
- Collar stud abscess.
- Cystic hygroma.
- Branchial cyst.
- Parotitis.

Congenital
- Thyroglossal duct cyst.
- Dermoid cyst.
- Torticollis.

Vascular
- Subclavian aneurysm.
- Subclavian ectasia.

Important diagnostic features

Children

Congenital and inflammatory lesions are common.
- Cystic hygroma: in infants, base of the neck, brilliant transillumination, 'come and go'.
- Thyroglossal or dermoid cyst: midline, discrete, elevates with tongue protrusion.
- Torticollis: rock-hard mass, more prominent with head flexed, associated with fixed rotation (a fibrous mass in the sternocleidomastoid muscle).
- Branchial cyst: anterior to the upper third of the sternocleidomastoid.
- Viral/bacterial adenitis: usually affects jugular nodes, multiple, tender masses.
- Neoplasms are unusual in children (lymphoma most common).

Young adults

Inflammatory neck masses and thyroid malignancy are common.
- Viral (e.g. infectious mononucleosis) or bacterial (tonsillitis/pharyngitis) adenitis.
- Papillary thyroid cancer: isolated, non-tender, thyroid mass, possible lymphadenopathy.

Over-40s

Neck lumps are malignant until proven otherwise.
- Metastatic lymphadenopathy: multiple, rock-hard, non-tender, tendency to be fixed.
- 75% in primary head and neck (thyroid, nasopharynx, tonsils, larynx, pharynx), 25% from infraclavicular primary (stomach, pancreas, lung).
- Primary lymphadenopathy (thyroid, lymphoma): fleshy, matted, rubbery, large size.
- Primary neoplasm (thyroid, salivary tumour): firm, non-tender, fixed to tissue of origin.

KEY INVESTIGATIONS

All patients–FBC
↓

?Thyroid	LAD	Primary tumours
• U/S scan: Solid/cystic.	• Full examination: Fundoscopy	• U/S scan.
• FNAC: Colloid nodule Follicular neoplasm Papillary carcinoma Anaplastic carcinoma.	Auroscopy Nasopharyngoscopy Laryngoscopy Bronchoscopy Gastroscopy.	• FNAC.
	• FNAC: ?Lymphoma/carcinoma.	
	• Biopsy: ?Lymphoma cell type.	
	• CXR	
	• CT scan: Source of carcinoma.	

---

2 Dysphagia

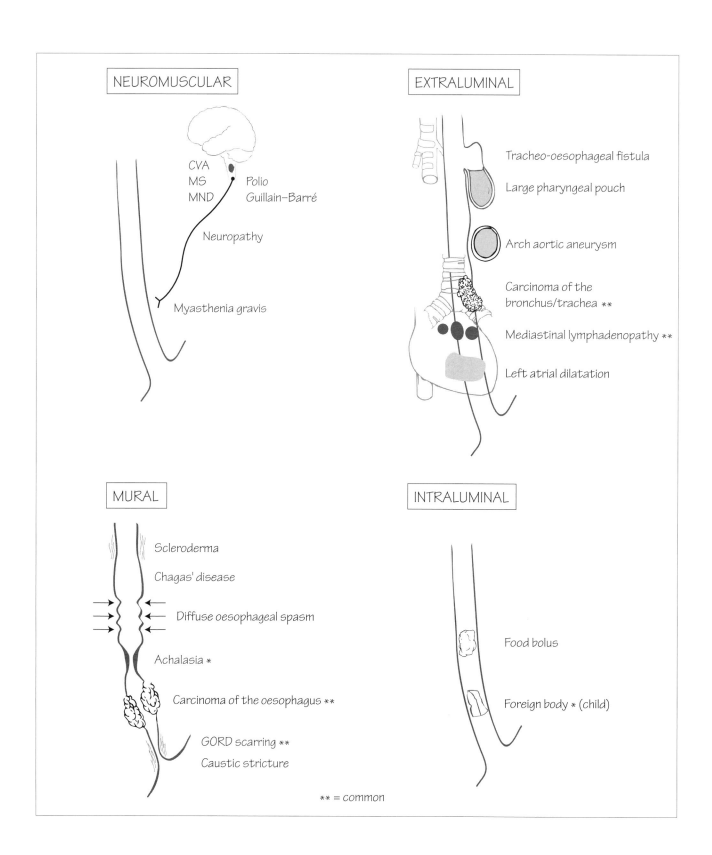

NEUROMUSCULAR

CVA
MS   Polio
MND   Guillain–Barré

Neuropathy

Myasthenia gravis

EXTRALUMINAL

Tracheo-oesophageal fistula

Large pharyngeal pouch

Arch aortic aneurysm

Carcinoma of the
bronchus/trachea **

Mediastinal lymphadenopathy **

Left atrial dilatation

MURAL

Scleroderma

Chagas' disease

Diffuse oesophageal spasm

Achalasia *

Carcinoma of the oesophagus **

GORD scarring **
Caustic stricture

INTRALUMINAL

Food bolus

Foreign body * (child)

** = common

Definition

Dysphagia literally means difficulty with swallowing, which may be associated with ingestion of solids or liquids or both.

Important diagnostic features

Mural

- Carcinoma of the oesophagus: progressive course, associated weight loss and anorexia, low-grade anaemia, possible small haematemesis.
- Reflux oesophagitis and stricture: preceded by heartburn, progressive course, nocturnal regurgitation.
- Achalasia: onset in young adulthood or old age, liquids disproportionately difficult to swallow, frequent regurgitation, recurrent chest infections, long history.
- Tracheo-oesophageal fistula-recurrent chest infections, coughing after drinking. Present in childhood (congenital) or late adulthood (post trauma, deep X-ray therapy (DXT) or malignant).
- Chagas' disease (*Trypanosoma cruzi*): South American prevalence, associated with dysrhythmias and colonic dysmotility.

- Caustic stricture: examination shows corrosive ingestion, chronic dysphagia, onset may be months after.
- Scleroderma: slow onset, associated with skin and hair changes.

Intraluminal

Foreign body: acute onset, marked retrosternal discomfort, dysphagia even to saliva is characteristic.

Extramural

- Pulsion diverticulum: intermittent symptoms, unexpected regurgitation.
- External compression: mediastinal lymph nodes, left atrial hypertrophy, bronchial malignancy.

KEY INVESTIGATIONS

All

FBC: anaemia (tumours much more commonly cause this than reflux).
LFTs: (hepatic disease).
↓

OGD
(moderate risk, specialist, good for differentiating tumour vs. achalasia vs. reflux stricture, allows biopsy for tissue diagnosis, allows possible treatment).

Barium swallow
(low risk, easy, good for possible fistula, high tumour, diverticulum, reflux).
↓

If ?dysmotility	If ?extrinsic compression
• achalasia	↓
• neurogenic causes	CXR (AP and lateral)
↓	CT scan: low risk, good for
Video barium swallow	extrinsic compression,
Oesophageal manometry	allows tumour staging

3 Haemoptysis

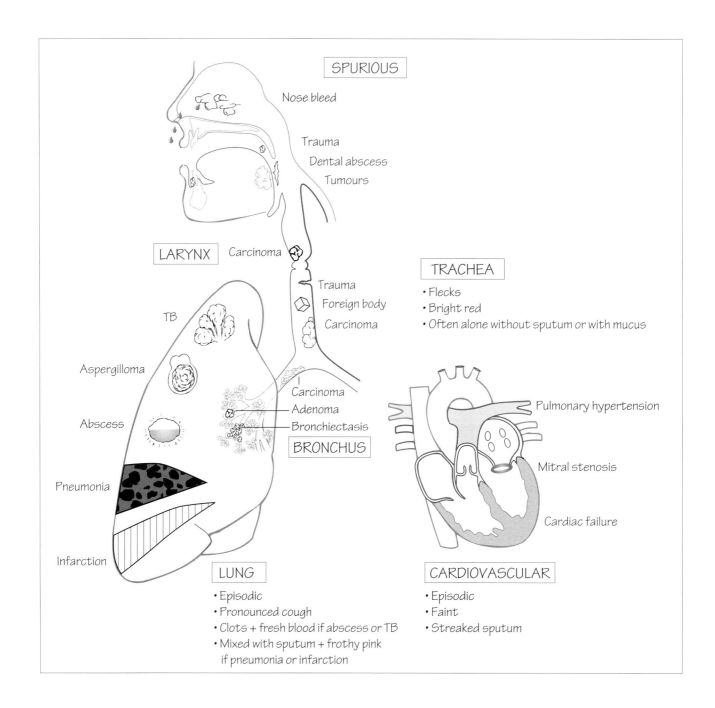

SPURIOUS

Nose bleed

Trauma
Dental abscess
Tumours

LARYNX

Carcinoma

TRACHEA
• Flecks
• Bright red
• Often alone without sputum or with mucus

Trauma
Foreign body
Carcinoma

TB

Aspergilloma

Abscess

Carcinoma
Adenoma
Bronchiectasis
BRONCHUS

Pulmonary hypertension

Mitral stenosis

Cardiac failure

Pneumonia

Infarction

LUNG
• Episodic
• Pronounced cough
• Clots + fresh blood if abscess or TB
• Mixed with sputum + frothy pink
  if pneumonia or infarction

CARDIOVASCULAR
• Episodic
• Faint
• Streaked sputum

Definition

Haemoptysis (blood spitting) is the symptom of coughing up blood from the lungs. Blood from the nose, mouth or pharynx that may also be spat out is termed 'spurious haemoptysis'.

KEY POINTS
- Blood from the proximal bronchi or trachea is usually bright red. It may be frankly blood or mixed with mucus and debris, particularly from a tumour.
- Blood from the distal bronchioles and alveoli is often pink and mixed with frothy sputum.

Important diagnostic features

The sources, causes and features are listed below.

Spurious haemoptysis

Mouth and nose
- Blood dyscrasias: associated nose bleeds, spontaneous bruising.
- Scurvy (vitamin C deficiency): poor hair/teeth, skin bruising.
- Dental caries, trauma, gingivitis.
- Oral tumours: painful intraoral mass, discharge, fetor.
- Hypertensive/spontaneous: no warning, brief bleed, often recurrent.
- Nasal tumours (common in South-East Asia).

True haemoptysis

Larynx and trachea
- Foreign body: choking, stridor, pain.
- Carcinoma: hoarse voice, bovine cough.

Bronchus
- Carcinoma: spontaneous haemoptysis, chest infections, weight loss, monophonic wheezing.
- Adenoma (e.g. carcinoid): recurrent chest infections, carcinoid syndrome.
- Bronchiectasis: chronic chest infections, fetor, blood mixed with purulent sputum, physical examination shows TB or severe chest infections.
- Foreign body: recurrent chest infections, sudden-onset inexplicable 'asthma'.

Lung
- TB: weight loss, fevers, night sweats, dry or productive cough.
- Pneumonia/lung abscess: features of acute chest sepsis, swinging fever.
- Pulmonary infarct (secondary to PE): pleuritic chest pain, tachypnoea, pleural rub.
- Aspergilloma.

Cardiac
- Mitral stenosis: frothy pink sputum, recurrent chest infections.
- LVF: frothy pink sputum, pulmonary oedema.

KEY INVESTIGATIONS

All
- Clotting: blood dyscrasias.
- FBC: infections, dyscrasias.
- Chest X-ray (AP and lateral).

↓

?Foreign body	?Cardiac cause	?Tumour	?Infection	?Infarction/PE
Bronchoscopy.	ECG	Sputum cytology	Sputum MC+S	V/Q scan
	Echocardiography.	CT scan	?CT scan.	CT scan.
		Bronchoscopy.		

4 Breast lump

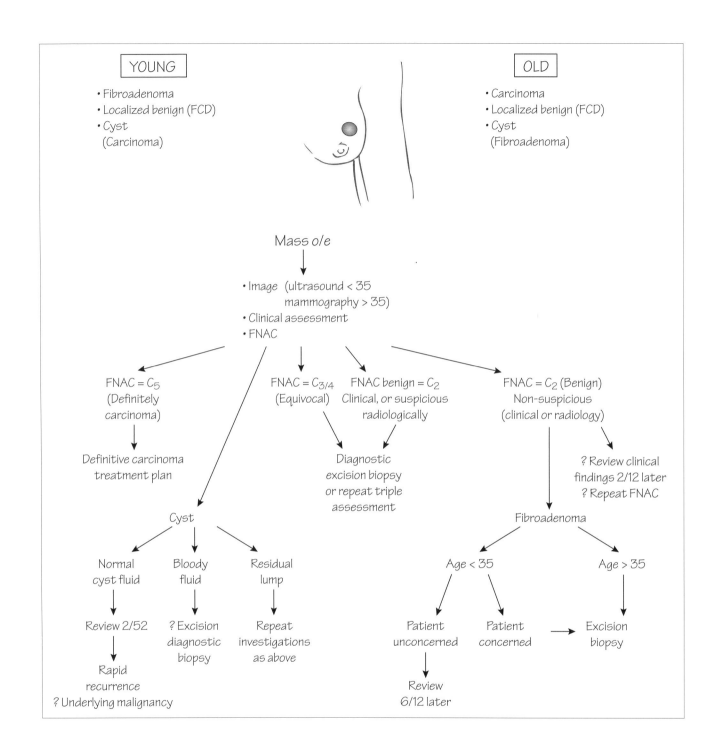

YOUNG
- Fibroadenoma
- Localized benign (FCD)
- Cyst
  (Carcinoma)

OLD
- Carcinoma
- Localized benign (FCD)
- Cyst
  (Fibroadenoma)

Mass o/e

- Image (ultrasound < 35
  mammography > 35)
- Clinical assessment
- FNAC

FNAC = C_5
(Definitely
carcinoma)

FNAC = $C_{3/4}$
(Equivocal)

FNAC benign = C_2
Clinical, or suspicious
radiologically

FNAC = C_2 (Benign)
Non-suspicious
(clinical or radiology)

Definitive carcinoma
treatment plan

Diagnostic
excision biopsy
or repeat triple
assessment

? Review clinical
findings 2/12 later
? Repeat FNAC

Cyst

Fibroadenoma

Normal
cyst fluid

Bloody
fluid

Residual
lump

Age < 35

Age > 35

Review 2/52

? Excision
diagnostic
biopsy

Repeat
investigations
as above

Patient
unconcerned

Patient
concerned

Excision
biopsy

Rapid
recurrence
? Underlying malignancy

Review
6/12 later

Definition

A breast lump is defined as any palpable mass in the breast. A breast lump is the most common presentation of both benign and malignant breast disease. Enlargement of the whole breast can occur either uni- or bilaterally, but this is not strictly a breast lump.

KEY POINTS
- The commonest breast lumps occurring under the age of 35 years are fibroadenomas and fibrocystic disease.
- The commonest breast lumps occurring over the age of 50 years are carcinomas and cysts.
- Pain is more characteristic of infection/inflammation than tumours.
- Skin/chest wall tethering is more characteristic of tumours than benign disease.
- Multiple lesions are usually benign (cysts or fibrocystic disease).

Differential diagnosis

Swelling of the whole breast

Bilateral
- Pregnancy, lactation.
- Idiopathic hypertrophy.
- Drug induced (e.g. stilboestrol, cimetidine).

Unilateral
- Enlargement in the newborn.
- Puberty.

Localized swellings in the breast

Mastitis/breast abscess
- During lactation: red, hot, tender lump, systemic upset.
- Tuberculous abscess: chronic, 'cold', recurrent, discharging sinus.

Cysts
- Galactocele: commoner postpartum, tender but not inflamed, milky contents.
- Fibrocystic disease: irregular, ill defined, often tender.

Solid lumps
Benign include:
- Fibroadenoma: discrete, firm, well defined, regular, highly mobile.
- Fat necrosis: irregular, ill defined, hard, ?skin tethering.
- Lipoma: well defined, soft, non-tender, fairly mobile.
- Cystosarcoma phylloides: wide surgical excision (10% are malignant).

Malignant include:
- Carcinoma
  early: ill defined, hard, irregular, skin tethering
  late: spreading fixity, ulceration, fungation, '*peau d'orange*'.

Swellings behind the breast
- Rib deformities, chondroma, costochondritis (Tietze's disease).

KEY INVESTIGATIONS
- FNAC: tumours, fibroadenoma, fibrocystic disease, fat necrosis, mastitis.
- Ultrasound: fibroadenoma, cysts, tumours (best for young women/ dense breasts).
- Mammography: tumours, cysts, fibrocystic disease, fat necrosis.
- Biopsy ('Trucut'/open surgical): usually provides definitive histology (may be radiologically guided if lump is small or impalpable—detected by mammography as part of breast screening programme).

5 Breast pain

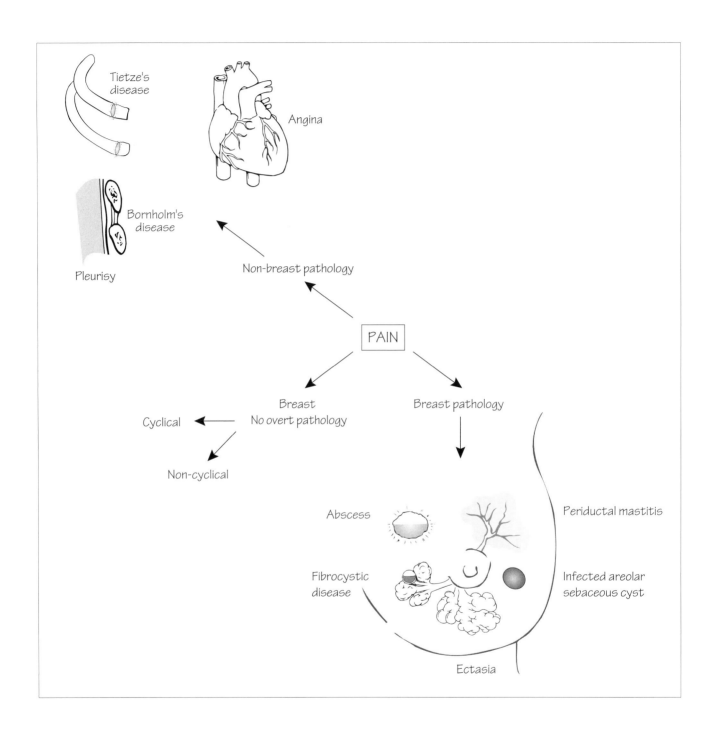

Definition

Mastalgia is any pain felt in the breast. *Cyclical mastalgia* is pain in the breast which varies in association with the menstrual cycle. *Non-cyclical mastalgia* is pain in the breast which follows no pattern or is intermittent.

KEY POINTS
- Mastalgia is commonly due to disorders of the breast or nipple tissue but may also be due to problems in the underlying chest wall or overlying skin.
- Pain is an uncommon presenting feature of tumours but any underlying mass should be investigated as for a mass (see Chapter 4).
- Always look for an associated infection in the breast.
- Mammography should be routine in women presenting over the age of 45 years to help exclude occult carcinoma.

Important diagnostic features

Non-breast conditions

- Tietze's disease (costochondritis): tenderness over medial ends of ribs, not limited to the breast area of the chest wall, relieved by NSAIDs.
- Bornholm's disease (epidemic pleurodynia): marked pain with no physical signs in the breast, worse with inspiration, no chest disease underlying, relieved with NSAIDs.
- Pleurisy: associated chest infection, pleural rub, may be bilateral.
- Angina: usually atypical angina, may be hard to diagnose, previous history of associated vascular disease.

Mastalgia due to breast pathology

Mastitis/breast abscess
- During lactation: red, hot, tender lump, systemic upset.
  Treatment: aspirate abscess (may need to be repeated), do not stop breast feeding, oral antibiotics.

- Non-lactational abscesses: recurrent, associated with smoking, associated with underlying ductal ectasia.
  Treatment: aspirate or incise and drain abscess, give oral antibiotics, stop smoking, prophylactic metronidazole for recurrent sepsis.

Infected sebaceous cyst
Single lump superficially in the skin of the periareolar region, previous history of painless cystic lump.
  Treatment: excise infected cyst.

Fibrocystic disease
Irregular, ill defined, may be associated lumps, tender more than very painful.

Mastalgia without breast pathology

- Pain often felt throughout the breast, often worse in the axillary tail, moderately tender to examination.
  Treatment for cyclical mastalgia: γ linoleic acid (evening primrose oil), danazol, tamoxifen.
  Treatment for non-cyclical mastalgia: NSAIDs, γ linoleic acid.

KEY INVESTIGATIONS
Non-breast origin
Chest X-ray, ECG (exercise)

Breast pathology
- FNAC (MC+S): associated palpable lump, ?fibrocystic disease, ?mastitis/abscess.
- Ultrasound (young women/dense breasts) or mammography (older women/small breasts).

Mastalgia without breast pathology
Mammography in women over 45 years

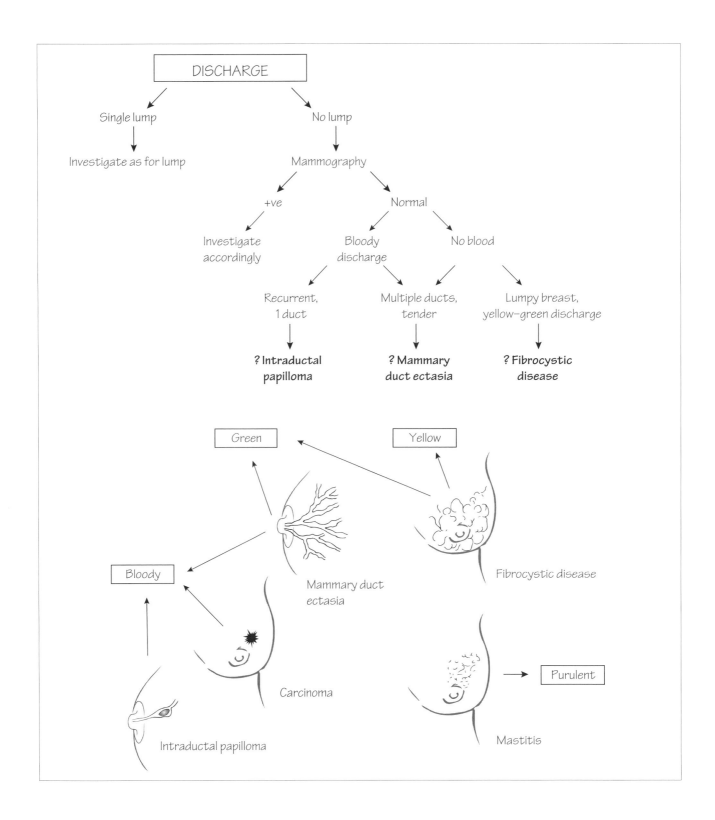

Definition

Any fluid (which may be physiological or pathological) emanating from the nipple.

Differential diagnosis

Physiological discharges

Milky or clear

- Lactation.
- Lactorrhoea in the newborn ('witches' milk').
- Lactorrhoea at puberty (may be in either sex).

Pathological discharges

Serous yellow-green

- Fibrocystic disease: cyclical, tender, lumpy breasts.

- Mammary duct ectasia: usually multiple ducts, intermittent, may be associated with low-grade mastitis.

Bloody

- Duct papilloma: single duct, ?retro-areolar, 'pea-sized' lump.
- Carcinoma: ?palpable lump.
- Mammary duct ectasia: usually multiple ducts, intermittent, may be associated with low-grade mastitis.

Pus ± milk

- Acute suppurative mastitis: tender, swollen, hot breast, multiple ducts discharging.
- Tuberculous (rare): chronic discharge, periareolar fistulae, 'sterile' cultures on normal media.

KEY INVESTIGATIONS

- MC+S: acute mastitis, TB (Lowenstein–Jensen medium, Ziehl–Neelsen stains).
- Discharge cytology: carcinoma.
- Mammography: tumours, fibrocystic disease, ?ectasia.
- Ductal excision: may be needed for exclusion of neoplasia.

7 Haematemesis

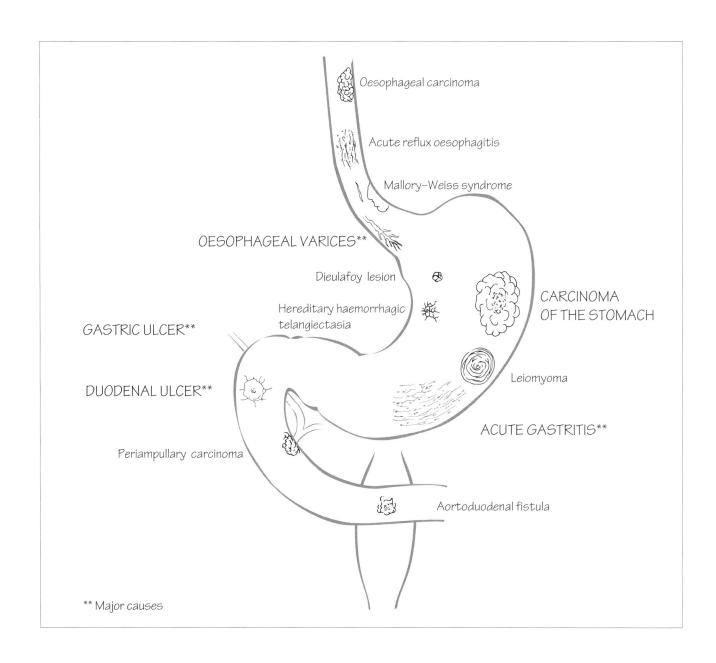

Oesophageal carcinoma

Acute reflux oesophagitis

Mallory–Weiss syndrome

OESOPHAGEAL VARICES**

Dieulafoy lesion

Hereditary haemorrhagic
telangiectasia

GASTRIC ULCER**

DUODENAL ULCER**

CARCINOMA
OF THE STOMACH

Leiomyoma

ACUTE GASTRITIS**

Periampullary carcinoma

Aortoduodenal fistula

** Major causes

Definitions

GI bleeding is any blood loss from the GI tract (from the mouth to the anus), which may present with haematemesis, melaena, rectal bleeding or anaemia. *Haematemesis* is defined as vomiting blood and is usually caused by upper GI disease. *Melaena* is the passage PR of a black treacle-like stool that contains altered blood, usually as a result of proximal bowel bleeding.

KEY POINTS

- Haematemesis is usually caused by lesions proximal to the duodeno-jejunal junction.
- Melaena may be caused by lesions anywhere from oesophagus to colon (upper GI lesions can cause frank PR bleeding).
- Most tumours more commonly cause anaemia than frank haematemesis.
- In young adults, peptic ulcer disease (PUD), congenital lesions and varices are common causes.
- In the elderly, tumours, PUD and angiodysplasia are common causes.

Important diagnostic features

Oesophagus

- Reflux oesophagitis: small volumes, bright red, associated with regurgitation.
- Oesophageal carcinoma (rare): scanty, blood-stained debris, rarely significant volume, associated with weight loss, anergia, dysphagia.
- Bleeding varices: sudden onset, painless, large volumes, dark red blood, history of (alcoholic) liver disease, physical findings of portal hypertension.
- Trauma during vomiting (Mallory–Weiss syndrome): bright red bloody vomit usually preceded by several normal but forceful vomiting episodes.

Stomach

- Erosive gastritis: small volumes, bright red, may follow alcohol or NSAID intake/stress, history of dyspeptic symptoms.
- Gastric ulcer: often larger-sized bleed, painless, possible herald smaller bleeds, accompanied by altered blood ('coffee grounds'), history of PUD.
- Gastric cancer: rarely large bleed, anaemia commoner, associated weight loss, anorexia, dyspeptic symptoms.
- Gastric leiomyoma (rare): spontaneous-onset moderate-sized bleed.
- Dieulafoy's disease (rare): younger patients, spontaneous large bleed, difficult to diagnose.

Duodenum

- Duodenal ulcer: past history of duodenal ulcer, melaena often also prominent, symptoms of back pain, hunger pains, NSAID use.
- Aortoduodenal fistula (rare): usually infected graft post AAA repair, massive haematemesis and PR bleed, usually fatal.

KEY INVESTIGATIONS

- FBC: carcinomas, reflux oesophagitis.
- LFTs: liver disease (varices).
- Clotting: alcohol, bleeding diatheses.
- OGD: investigation of choice. High diagnostic accuracy, allows therapeutic manoeuvres also (varices: injection; ulcers: injection/cautery).
- Angiography: rare duodenal causes, obscure recurrent bleeds.
- Barium meal and follow through: useful for patients who are unfit for OGD (respiratory disease) and ?proximal jejunal lesions.

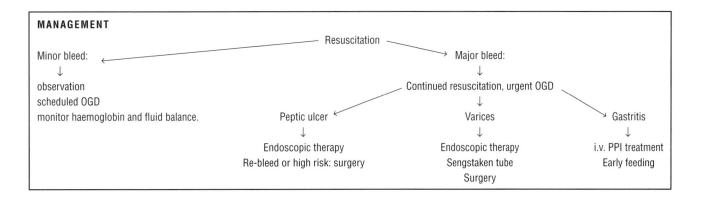

MANAGEMENT

Resuscitation

Minor bleed: → observation, scheduled OGD, monitor haemoglobin and fluid balance.

Major bleed: → Continued resuscitation, urgent OGD

- Peptic ulcer → Endoscopic therapy; Re-bleed or high risk: surgery
- Varices → Endoscopic therapy; Sengstaken tube; Surgery
- Gastritis → i.v. PPI treatment; Early feeding

8 Dyspepsia

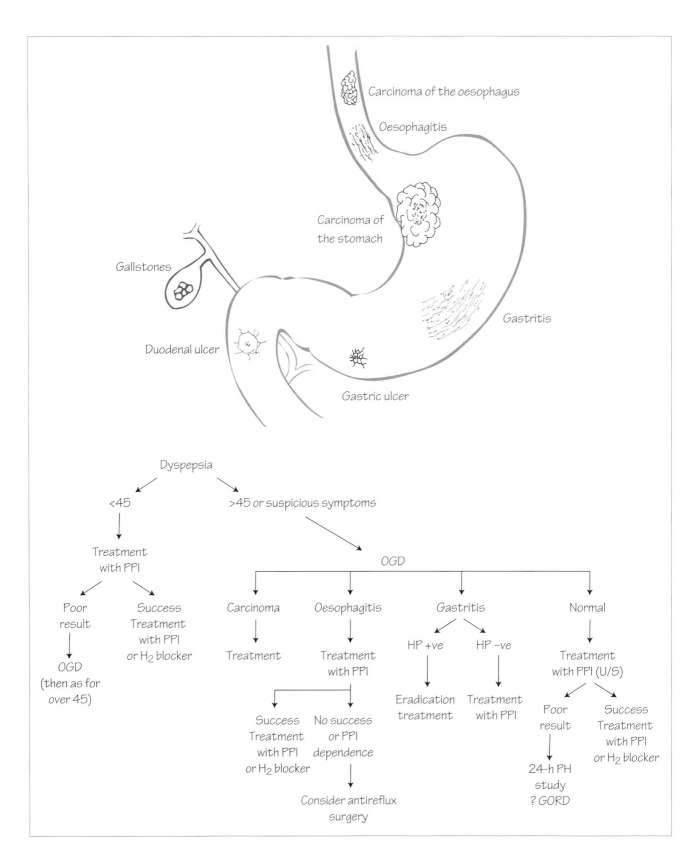

Definition

Dyspepsia is the feeling of discomfort or pain in the upper abdomen or lower chest. *Indigestion* may be used by the patient to mean dyspepsia, regurgitation symptoms or flatulence.

> **KEY POINTS**
> • Dyspepsia may be the only presenting symptom of upper GI malignancy. All older patients and patients with atypical history should have endoscopy.
> • In young adults, gastro-oesophageal reflux and *Helicobacter*-positive gastritis are common causes.
> • Dyspepsia is rarely the only symptom of gallstones—they are more often incidental findings.

Differential diagnosis

Oesophagus

• Reflux oesophagitis: retrosternal dyspepsia, worse after large meal/lying down, associated symptoms of regurgitation, pain on swallowing.
• Oesophageal carcinoma: new-onset dyspepsia in older patient, associated symptoms of weight loss/dysphagia/haematemesis, failure to respond to acid suppression treatment.

Stomach

• Gastritis: recurrent episodes of epigastric pain, transient or short-lived symptoms, may be associated with diet, responds well to antacids/acid suppression.

• Gastric ulcer: typically chronic epigastric pain, worse with food, 'food fear' may lead to weight loss, exacerbated by smoking/alcohol, occasionally relieved by vomiting.
• Carcinoma stomach: progressive symptoms, associated weight loss/anorexia, iron-deficient anaemia common, early satiety, epigastric mass.

Duodenum

• Duodenal ulcer: epigastric and back pain, chronic exacerbations lasting several weeks, relieved by food especially milky drinks, relieved by bed rest, commoner in younger men, associated with *Helicobacter* infection.
• Duodenitis: often transient, mild symptoms only, associated with alcohol and smoking.

Gallstones

Dyspepsia is rarely the only symptom, associated RUQ pain, needs normal OGD and positive ultrasound to be considered as cause for dyspeptic symptoms.

> **KEY INVESTIGATIONS**
> • FBC: anaemia suggests malignancy.
> • OGD: tumours, PUD, assessment of oesophagitis.
> • 24-hour pH monitoring: ?GORD.
> • Ultrasound: ?gallstones.

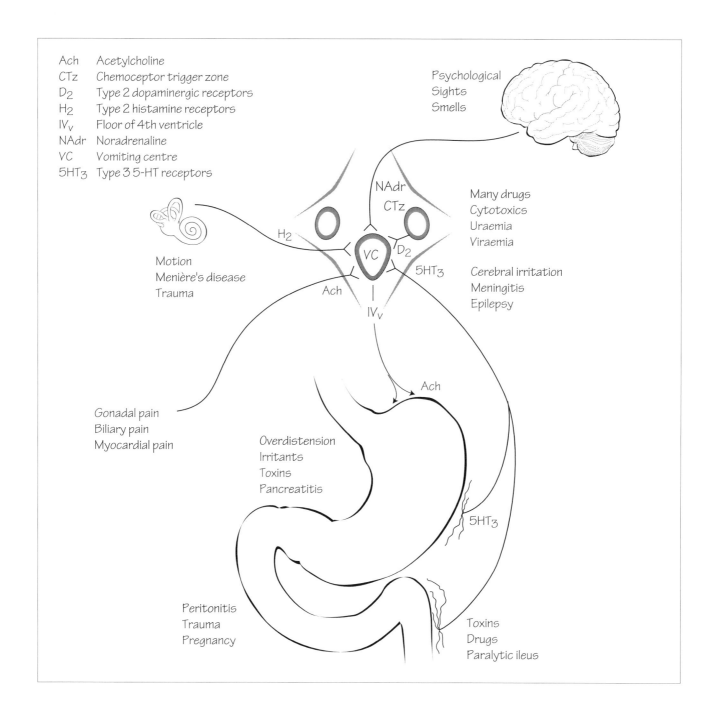

Ach   Acetylcholine
CTz   Chemoceptor trigger zone
D_2 Type 2 dopaminergic receptors
H_2 Type 2 histamine receptors
IV_v Floor of 4th ventricle
NAdr   Noradrenaline
VC   Vomiting centre
$5HT_3$ Type 3 5-HT receptors

Psychological
Sights
Smells

NAdr
CTz

H_2

VC

D_2

$5HT_3$

Many drugs
Cytotoxics
Uraemia
Viraemia

Cerebral irritation
Meningitis
Epilepsy

Motion
Menière's disease
Trauma

Ach

IV_v

Ach

Gonadal pain
Biliary pain
Myocardial pain

Overdistension
Irritants
Toxins
Pancreatitis

$5HT_3$

Peritonitis
Trauma
Pregnancy

Toxins
Drugs
Paralytic ileus

Definitions

Vomiting is defined as the involuntary return to, and forceful expulsion from, the mouth of all or part of the contents of the stomach. *Waterbrash* is the sudden secretion and accumulation of saliva in the mouth as a reflex associated with dyspepsia. *Retching* is the process whereby forceful contractions of the diaphragm and abdominal muscles occur without evacuation of the stomach contents.

> **KEY POINTS**
> • Vomiting is initiated when the vomiting centre in the medulla oblongata is stimulated, either directly (central vomiting) or via various afferent fibres (reflex vomiting).
> • Vomiting of different origins is mediated by different pathways and transmitters. Therapy is best directed according to cause.
> • Consider mechanical causes (e.g. gastric outflow or intestinal obstruction) before starting therapy.

Important diagnostic features

Central vomiting
- Drugs, e.g. morphine sulphate, chemotherapeutic agents.
- Uraemia.
- Viral hepatitis.
- Hypercalcaemia of any cause.
- Acute infections, especially in children.
- Pregnancy.

Reflex vomiting

Gastrointestinal causes (5HT3 and Ach mediated— treatment: promotilants, 5HT3 antagonists)
- Ingestion of irritants.
  Bacteria, e.g. salmonella (gastroenteritis).
  Emetics, e.g. zinc sulphate, ipecacuanha.
  Drugs, e.g. alcohol, salicylates (gastritis).
  Poisons, e.g. salt, arsenic, phosphorus.

- PUD: especially gastric ulcer; vomiting relieves the pain.
- Intestinal obstruction.
  Hour-glass stomach (carcinoma of the stomach).
  Pyloric stenosis—infant: hypertrophic pyloric stenosis, projectile vomiting; adult: pyloric outlet obstruction secondary to PUD or malignant disease.
  Small bowel obstruction: adhesions, hernia, neoplasm, Crohn's disease.
  Large bowel obstruction: malignancy, volvulus, diverticular disease.
- Inflammation: appendicitis, peritonitis, pancreatitis, cholecystitis, biliary colic.

General causes (ACh and D2 mediated—treatment: anticholinergics, antidopaminergics)
- Myocardial infarction.
- Ovarian disease, ectopic pregnancy.
- Severe pain (e.g. kick to the testis, gonadal torsion, blow to the epigastrium).
- Severe coughing (e.g. pulmonary TB, pertussis).

CNS causes (NAdr and ACh mediated—treatment: anticholinergics, sedatives)
- Raised intracranial pressure.
  Head injury.
  Cerebral tumour or abscess.
  Hydrocephalus.
  Meningitis.
  Cerebral haemorrhage.
- Migraine.
- Epilepsy.
- Offensive sights, tastes and smells.
- Hysteria.
- Middle ear disorders (H_2 mediated—treatment: antihistamines).
  Menière's disease.
  Travel/motion sickness.

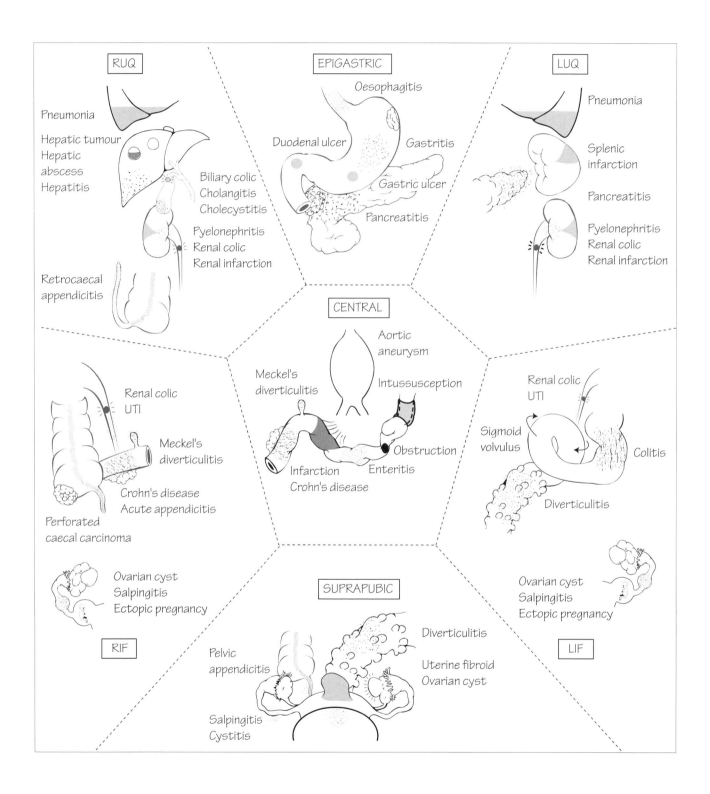

Definitions

Abdominal pain is a subjective unpleasant sensation felt in any of the abdominal regions. *Acute* abdominal pain is usually used to refer to pain of sudden onset, and/or short duration. *Referred pain* is the perception of pain in an area remote from the site of origin of the pain.

KEY POINTS

- The level of abdominal pain generally relates to the origin: foregut—upper; midgut—middle; hindgut—lower.
- Generally, colicky (visceral) pain is caused by stretching or contracting a hollow viscus (e.g. gallbladder, ureter, ileum).
- Generally, constant localized (somatic) pain is caused by peritoneal irritation and indicates the presence of inflammation/infection (e.g. pancreatitis, cholecystitis, appendicitis).
- Associated back pain suggests retroperitoneal pathology (aortic aneurysm, pancreatitis, posterior DU, pyelonephritis).
- Associated sacral or perineal pain suggests pelvic pathology (ovarian cyst, PID, pelvic abscess).
- Generally, very severe pain indicates ischaemia or generalized peritonitis (e.g. mesenteric infarction, perforated duodenal ulcer).
- Pain out of proportion to the physical signs suggests ischaemia without perforation.
- Remember referred causes of pain: pneumonia (right lower lobe), myocardial infarction, lumbar nerve root pathology.

KEY INVESTIGATIONS

- FBC: leucocytosis, infective/inflammatory diseases, anaemia, occult malignancy, PUD.
- LFTs: usually abnormal in cholangitis, may be abnormal in acute cholecystitis.
- Amylase: serum level >1000 iu diagnostic of pancreatitis. Serum level 500–1000 iu, ?pancreatitis, perforated ulcer, bowel ischaemia, severe sepsis. Serum level raised <500 iu, non-specific indicator of pathology.
- β-HCG (serum): ectopic pregnancy.
- Arterial blood gases: metabolic acidosis—?bowel ischaemia, peritonitis, pancreatitis.
- MSU: urinary tract infection (++ve nitrites, blood, protein), renal stone (++ve blood).
- ECG: myocardial infarction.
- Chest X-ray: perforated viscus (free gas), pneumonia.
- Abdominal X-ray:
  ischaemic bowel (dilated, thickened oedematous loops)
  pancreatitis ('sentinel' dilated upper jejunum)
  cholangitis (air in biliary tree)
  acute colitis (dilated, oedematous, featureless colon)
  acute obstruction (dilated loops, 'string of pearls' sign)
  renal stones (radiodense opacity in renal tract).
- Ultrasound:
  intra-abdominal abscesses (diverticular, appendicular, pelvic)
  acute cholecystitis/empyema
  ovarian pathology (cyst, ectopic pregnancy)
  trauma (liver/spleen haematoma)
  renal infections.
- OGD:
  PUD, gastritis.
- CT scan:
  pancreatitis, trauma (liver/spleen/mesenteric injuries), diverticulitis, leaking aortic aneurysm.
- IVU: renal stones, renal tract obstruction.

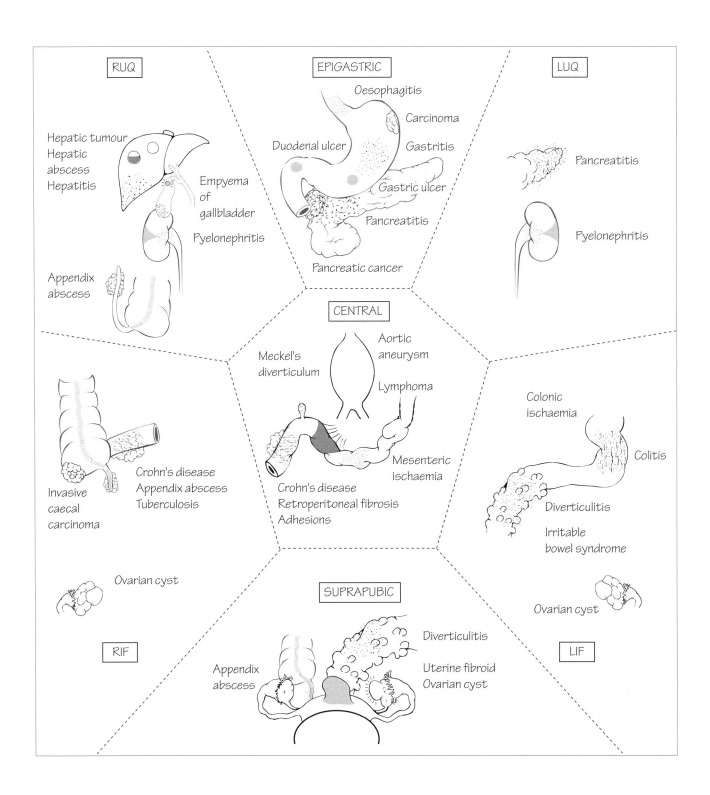

Definition

Chronic abdominal pain is usually used to refer to pain which is either longstanding, of prolonged duration or of recurrent/intermittent nature. Chronic pain may be associated with acute exacerbations.

Important diagnostic features

Irritable bowel syndrome

• Syndrome of colicky abdominal pain, bloating, hard pellety or watery stools, sensation of incomplete evacuation, often associated with frequency and urgency.
• Blood, mucus, abdominal physical findings, weight loss or recent onset of symptoms or onset in old age should suggest an organic cause and require thorough investigation.

Adhesions

• Associated with several syndromes of chronic or recurrent abdominal symptoms.
• **Adhesional abdominal pain**: difficult to diagnosis with any confidence, usually a diagnosis of exclusion, may be suggested by small bowel enema showing evidence of delayed transit or fixed strictures, rarely responds well to surgery.
• **Recurrent incomplete small bowel obstruction**: transient episodes of obstructive symptoms, often do not have all classical signs or symptoms present, abdominal signs may be unremarkable, self limiting.

Mesenteric angina

Classically occurs shortly after eating in elderly patients, colicky central abdominal pain, vomiting, food fear and weight loss. Usually associated with other occlusive vascular disease.

Meckel's diverticulum

May cause undiagnosed central abdominal pain in young adults. Occasionally associated with obscure PR bleeding, anaemia. Best diagnosed by radionuclide scanning.

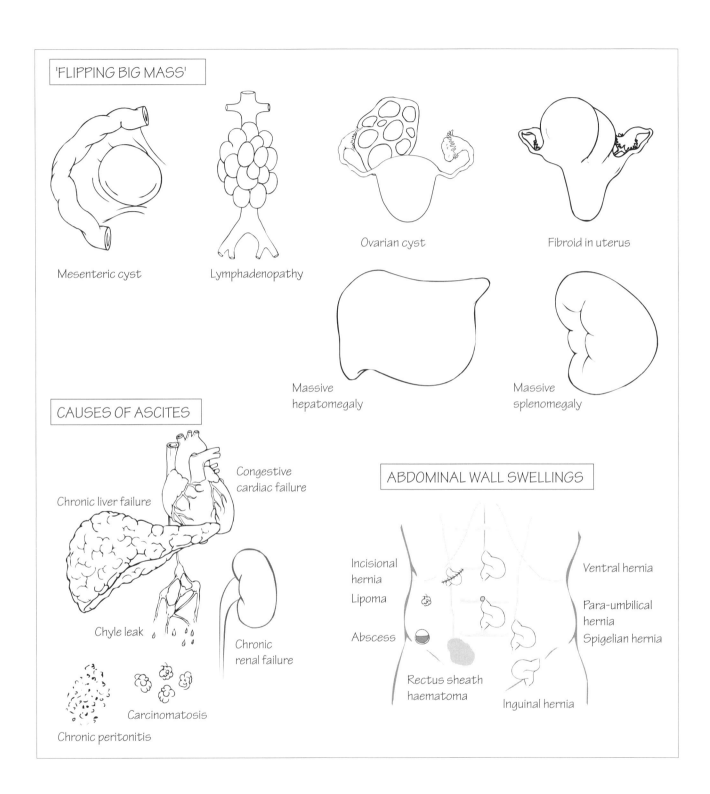

'FLIPPING BIG MASS'

Mesenteric cyst

Lymphadenopathy

Ovarian cyst

Fibroid in uterus

Massive hepatomegaly

Massive splenomegaly

CAUSES OF ASCITES

Chronic liver failure

Congestive cardiac failure

Chyle leak

Chronic renal failure

Carcinomatosis

Chronic peritonitis

ABDOMINAL WALL SWELLINGS

Incisional hernia

Lipoma

Abscess

Rectus sheath haematoma

Inguinal hernia

Ventral hernia

Para-umbilical hernia

Spigelian hernia

Definition

An abdominal swelling is an abnormal protuberance that arises from the abdominal cavity or the abdominal wall and may be general or localized, acute or chronic, cystic or solid.

> **KEY POINTS**
> - Generalized abdominal swellings affect the entire abdominal cavity.
> - Localized swellings can be located in the various regions of the abdomen.
> - Abdominal wall swellings can be differentiated from intra-abdominal swellings by asking the patient to raise his or her head from the couch (intraperitoneal swellings disappear while abdominal wall swellings persist).
> - Giant masses, other than ovarian cystadenocarcinoma, are rarely malignant.

Important diagnostic features

'Fat'

Obesity: deposition of fat in the abdominal wall and intra-abdominally (extraperitoneal layer, omentum and mesentery). Clinical obesity is present when a person's body weight is 120% greater than that recommended for their height, age and sex (body mass index).

'Flatus'

Intestinal obstruction: swallowed air accumulates in the bowel causing distension. This gives a tympanic note on percussion and produces the characteristic air-fluid levels and 'ladder' pattern on an abdominal radiograph. Sigmoid or caecal volvulus produces gross distension with characteristic features of distended loops on abdominal X-ray.

'Fluid'

- Intestinal obstruction: as well as air, fluid accumulates in the obstructed intestine.
- Ascites: fluid accumulates in the peritoneal cavity due to the '6 Cs':
  - chronic peritonitis (e.g. tuberculosis, missed appendicitis)
  - carcinomatosis (malignant deposits, especially ovary, stomach)
  - chronic liver disease (cirrhosis, secondary deposits, portal or hepatic vein obstruction, parasitic infections)
  - congestive heart failure (RVF)
  - chronic renal failure (nephrotic syndrome)
  - chyle (lymphatic duct disruption).

'Faeces'

Chronic constipation: faeces accumulate in the colon producing abdominal distension. Congenital causes include spina bifida and Hirschsprung's disease. Acquired causes include emotional disorders, chronic dehydration, drugs (opiates, anticholinergics, phenothiazines) and hypothyroidism.

'Fetus'

Pregnancy: swelling arises out of the pelvis.

'Flipping big mass'

Usually cystic lesions: giant ovarian cystadenoma, mesenteric cyst, retroperitoneal lymphadenopathy (lymphoma), giant uterine fibroid, giant splenomegaly, giant hepatomegaly, giant renal tumour, desmoid tumour.

> **KEY INVESTIGATIONS**
> - FBC: lymphomas, infections.
> - LFTs: liver disease.
> - U+Es: renal disease.
> - Abdominal X-ray:
>   ascites ('ground glass' appearance, loss of visceral outlines)
>   large mass (bowel gas pattern eccentric, paucity of gas in one quadrant)
>   fibroid ('popcorn' calcification).
> - Ultrasound: ascites, may show cystic masses.
> - CT scan: investigation of choice, differentiates origin and relationships.
> - Paracentesis: MC+S (infections), cytology (tumours).
> - Liver biopsy: undiagnosed hepatomegaly.

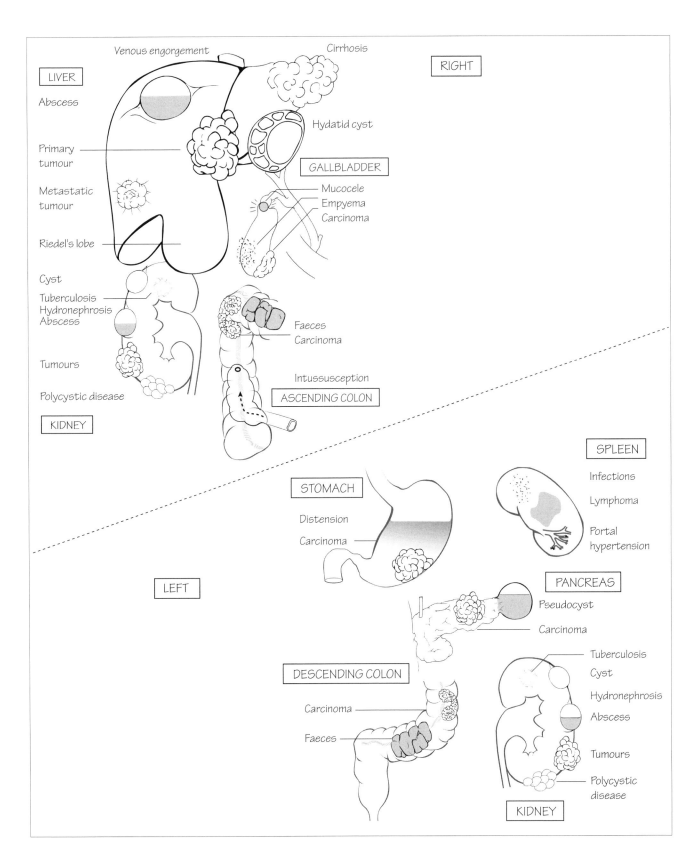

Liver

• Riedel's lobe: smooth, non-tender, lateral/right lobe:, 'tongue-like', men < women.
• Infective hepatitis: smooth, tender, global enlargement.
• Liver abscess: usually one large abscess, ?amoebic, very tender, systemically unwell.
• Hydatid cyst: smooth, may be loculated, ?history of tropical travel.
• Venous congestion: smooth, tender, pulsatile (slightly irregular (cirrhotic) if chronic).
• Cirrhosis: irregular, firm, 'knobbly'.
• Tumours:
  primary: solitary, large, non-tender, ?lobulated
  secondary: often multiple, irregular, rock hard, centrally umbilicated.

Gallbladder

• Generally: oval, smooth, projects towards RIF, beneath the tip of the ninth rib, moves with respiration.
• Mucocele: large gallbladder, moderately tender, smooth walled.
• Empyema: acutely tender, difficult to palpate clearly because of pain.
• Carcinoma of gallbladder: nodular, hard, irregular.

Renal masses

• Perinephric abscess/pyonephrosis: acutely tender, systemic signs, rarely large.
• Hydronephrosis: large, smooth, tense kidney. May be massive.
• Solitary cyst: smooth, non-tender, may be massive.
• Polycystic disease: frequently very large, lobulated, smooth.
• Renal carcinoma: irregular, nodular, often hard, ?fixed.
• Nephroblastoma: large mass in children.

Suprarenal gland

• Generally: only palpable when large, moves with respiration, difficult to define borders.
• Adenomas: usually cystic if palpable.
• Infections: ?chronic fungal infections, may be tender, systemic features.
• Congenital hyperplasia: young children, endocrine disorders associated, smooth, non-tender.

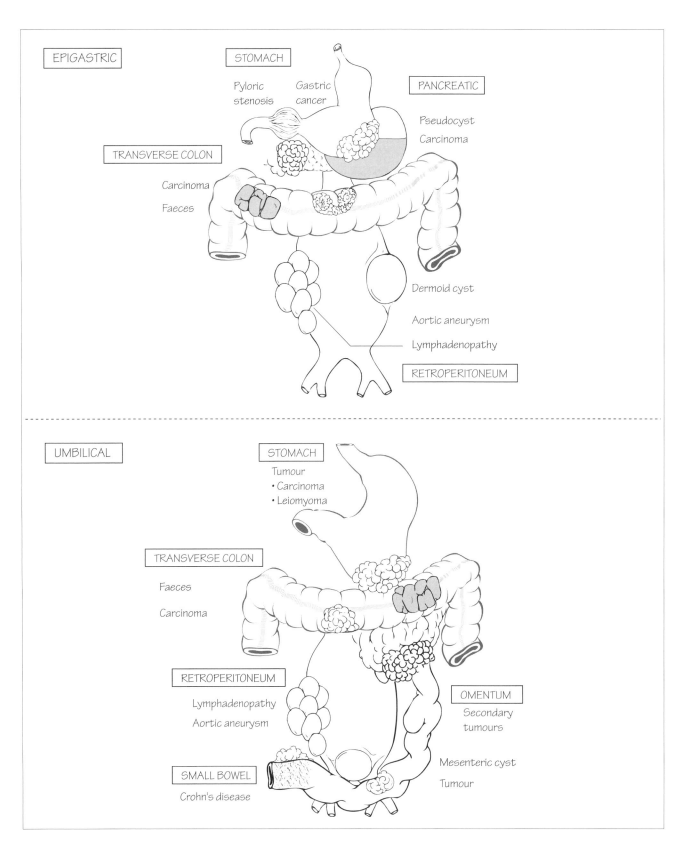

Colon

- Faeces: soft, putty-like mass, mobile, non-tender, can be indented.
- Carcinoma: firm–hard, irregular, non-tender, may be mobile (fixity strongly suggests carcinoma).
- Intussusception: mobile, smooth, sausage-shaped mass.

Stomach

- Gastric distension: soft, fluctuant, succussion splash present.
- Neoplasm: irregular, hard, craggy, immobile, does not descend on inspiration.

Pancreas

- Generally: does not move with respiration, fixed to retroperitoneum, poorly defined.
- Pseudocyst/cyst: mildly tender (worse if infected), symptoms of gastric obstruction.
- Carcinoma: hard, irregular, non-tender, fixed.

Retroperitoneum

- Lymphadenopathy: solid, immobile, irregular, 'rubbery', may be massive, particularly if lymphomatous.

- Dermoid cysts (rare): deep seated, smooth, recurrent after surgery.
- Aortic aneurysm: smooth, fusiform, pulsatile, expansile, may be tender.

Omentum

Secondary carcinoma: hard, irregular, mobile, 'pancake like', often ovarian carcinoma.

KEY INVESTIGATIONS

- FBC: anaemia—tumours.
- WCC: lymphomas, Crohn's disease, appendicitis/diverticulitis.
- LFTs: liver lesions.
- Ultrasound: pancreatic (pseudo)cysts, aortic aneurysm.
- CT scan: pancreatic tumours, lymphadenopathy, retroperitoneal/mesenteric cysts, aortic aneurysm, omental deposits.
- Gastroscopy: stomach tumours.
- Colonoscopy: colonic tumours.
- Small bowel enema: small intestinal tumours.
- Barium enema: colonic tumours.

14 Abdominal swellings (localized): lower abdominal

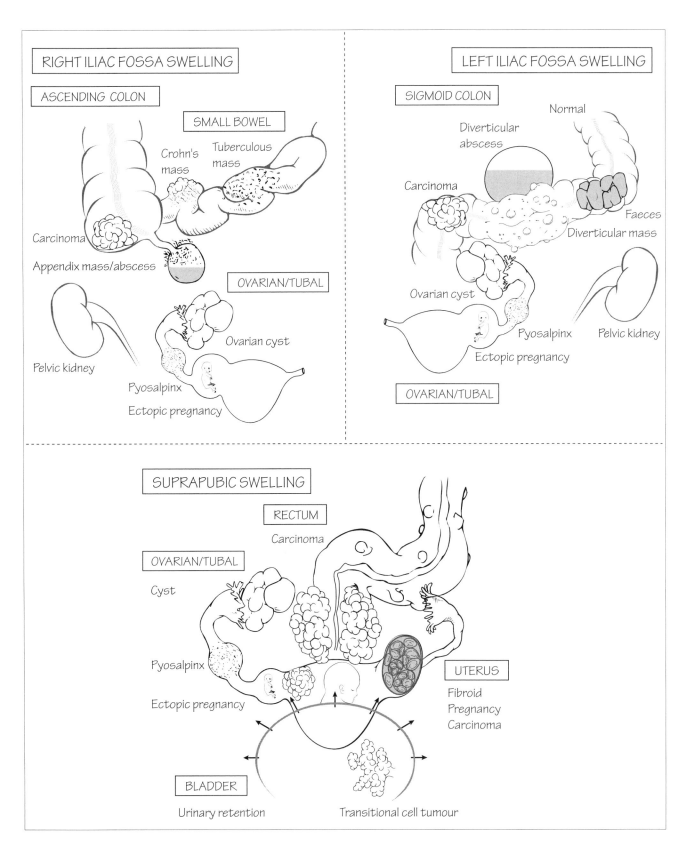

Sigmoid colon

- Diverticular mass: tender, ill defined, rubbery hard, non-mobile.
- Paracolic abscess: acutely tender, ill defined, ?fluctuant, systemic upset.
- Carcinoma: hard, craggy, non-tender unless perforated, immobile, associated with altered bowel habit/obstructive symptoms.
- Faeces: firm, indentable/'malleable', mobile with colon.
- Normal: only in a thin person, non-tender, chord like.

Caecum/ascending colon

- Appendix mass/abscess: acutely tender, ill defined, ?fluctuant, systemic upset.
- Carcinoma: hard, craggy, non-tender unless perforated, immobile, associated with anaemia/weight loss and anergia.

Terminal ileum

- Crohn's mass: tender, ill defined, rubbery hard, non-mobile.
- Tuberculous mass: mildly tender, ill defined, firm, associated with cutaneous sinuses, ?systemic TB.

Ovary/fallopian tube

- Cyst: may be massive, usually mobile, ?bimanually palpable on PV examination.
- Neoplasm.
- Ectopic pregnancy: very tender, associated with PV bleeding/intra-abdominal bleeding and collapse.
- Salpingo-oophoritis: very tender, bimanually palpable, associated with PV discharge.

Bladder

- Generally: midline swelling, extends up towards umbilicus, dull to percussion, non-mobile, cannot 'get below' it.
- Retention of urine: stony dull to percussion, associated with desire to pass urine, disappears on voiding/catheterization.
- Transitional cell carcinoma: hard, irregular, fixed, may be associated with dysuria, haematuria and desire to pass urine on examination.

Uterus

- Pregnancy: smooth, regular, fetal heart sounds heard/movements!
- Fibromyoma: usually smooth, may be pedunculated and mobile, non-tender, associated menorrhagia.
- Uterine carcinoma: firm uterus, may be tender, irregular only if tumour is extrauterine, associated PV bloody discharge.

Rectum

Carcinoma: firm, irregular, non-tender, relatively immobile, associated alteration in bowel habit/PR bleeding.

Urachus (rare)

Cyst: small swelling in midline, ?associated umbilical discharge.

Other

Pelvic kidney: smooth, regular, non-tender, non-mobile.

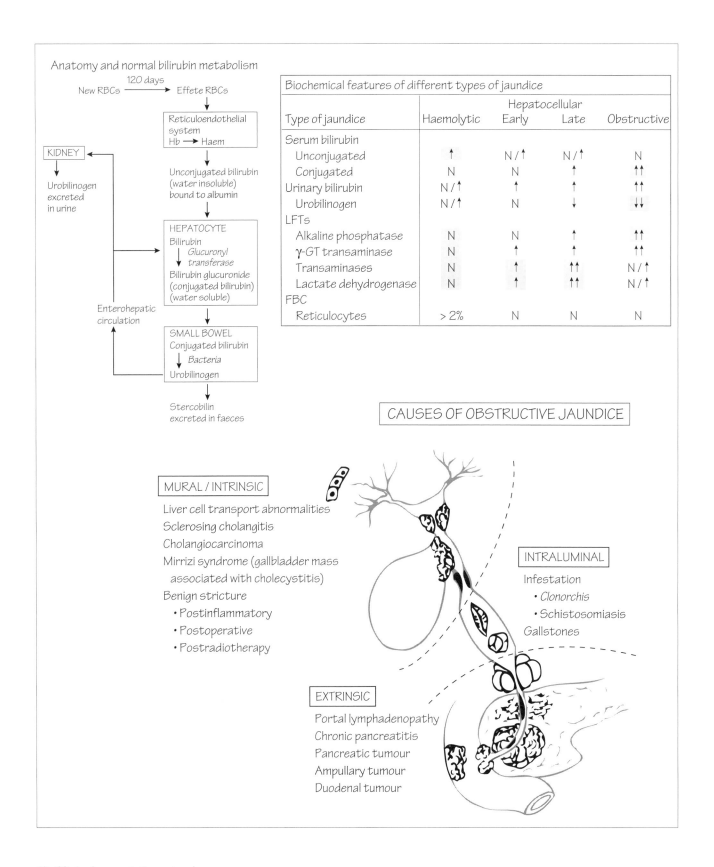

Anatomy and normal bilirubin metabolism

New RBCs → (120 days) → Effete RBCs

Reticuloendothelial system
Hb → Haem

KIDNEY

Urobilinogen excreted in urine

Unconjugated bilirubin (water insoluble) bound to albumin

HEPATOCYTE
Bilirubin
↓ *Glucuronyl transferase*
Bilirubin glucuronide (conjugated bilirubin) (water soluble)

Enterohepatic circulation

SMALL BOWEL
Conjugated bilirubin
↓ *Bacteria*
Urobilinogen

Stercobilin excreted in faeces

Biochemical features of different types of jaundice				
		Hepatocellular		
Type of jaundice	Haemolytic	Early	Late	Obstructive
Serum bilirubin				
Unconjugated	↑	N / ↑	N / ↑	N
Conjugated	N	N	↑	↑↑
Urinary bilirubin	N / ↑	↑	↑	↑↑
Urobilinogen	N / ↑	N	↓	↓↓
LFTs				
Alkaline phosphatase	N	N	↑	↑↑
γ-GT transaminase	N	↑	↑	↑↑
Transaminases	N	↑	↑↑	N / ↑
Lactate dehydrogenase	↑	↑	↑↑	N / ↑
FBC				
Reticulocytes	> 2%	N	N	N

CAUSES OF OBSTRUCTIVE JAUNDICE

MURAL / INTRINSIC

Liver cell transport abnormalities
Sclerosing cholangitis
Cholangiocarcinoma
Mirrizi syndrome (gallbladder mass associated with cholecystitis)
Benign stricture
• Postinflammatory
• Postoperative
• Postradiotherapy

INTRALUMINAL

Infestation
• *Clonorchis*
• *Schistosomiasis*
Gallstones

EXTRINSIC

Portal lymphadenopathy
Chronic pancreatitis
Pancreatic tumour
Ampullary tumour
Duodenal tumour

Definitions

Jaundice (also called icterus) is defined as yellowing of the skin and sclera from accumulation of the pigment bilirubin in the blood and tissues. The bilirubin level has to exceed 35–40 mmol/l before jaundice is clinically apparent.

> **KEY POINTS**
> - Jaundice can be classified simply as pre-hepatic (haemolytic), hepatic (hepatocellular) and post-hepatic (obstructive).
> - Most of the surgically treatable causes of jaundice are post-hepatic (obstructive).
> - Painless progressive jaundice is highly likely to be due to malignancy.

Differential diagnosis

The following list explains the mechanisms behind the causes of jaundice.

Pre-hepatic/haemolytic jaundice

Haemolytic/congenital hyperbilirubinaemias

Excess production of unconjugated bilirubin exhausts the capacity of the liver to conjugate the extra load, e.g. haemolytic anaemias (e.g. hereditary spherocytosis, sickle cell disease, hypersplenism, thalassaemia).

Hepatic/hepatocellular jaundice

Hepatic unconjugated hyperbilirubinaemia

- Failure of transport of unconjugated bilirubin into the cell, e.g. Gilbert's syndrome.
- Failure of glucuronyl transferase activity, e.g. Crigler–Najjar syndrome.

Hepatic conjugated hyperbilirubinaemia

Hepatocellular injury. Hepatocyte injury results in failure of excretion of bilirubin, e.g.

infections: viral hepatitis;

poisons: CCl_4, aflatoxin;

drugs: paracetamol, halothane.

Post-hepatic/obstructive jaundice

Post-hepatic conjugated hyperbilirubinaemia

Anything that blocks the release of conjugated bilirubin from the hepatocyte or prevents its delivery to the duodenum.

Courvoisier's law

'A palpable gallbladder in the presence of jaundice is unlikely to be due to gallstones.' It usually indicates the presence of a neoplastic stricture (tumour of pancreas, ampulla, duodenum, CBD), chronic pancreatitic stricture or portal lymphadenopathy.

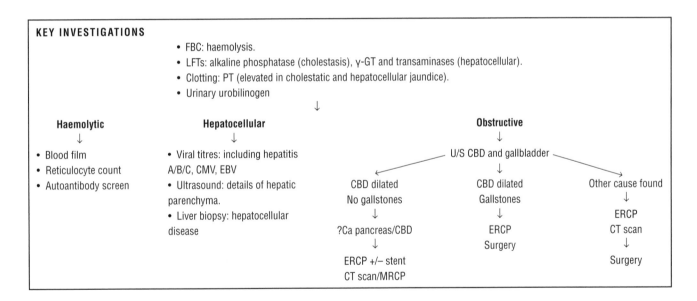

KEY INVESTIGATIONS

- FBC: haemolysis.
- LFTs: alkaline phosphatase (cholestasis), γ-GT and transaminases (hepatocellular).
- Clotting: PT (elevated in cholestatic and hepatocellular jaundice).
- Urinary urobilinogen

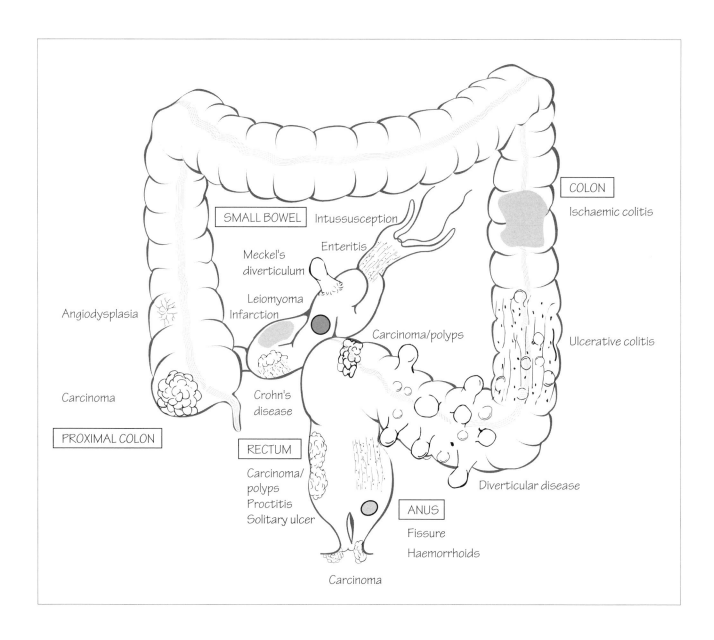

Important diagnostic features

Small intestine

• Meckel's diverticulum: young adults, painless bleeding, darker red/melaena common.

• Intussusception: young children, colicky abdominal pain, retching, bright red/mucus stool.

• Enteritis (infective/radiation/Crohn's).

• Ischaemic: severe abdominal pain, physical examination shows mesenteric ischaemia or AF, few signs, later collapse and shock.

• Tumours (leiomyoma/lymphoma): rare, intermittent history, often modest volumes lost.

Proximal colon

• Angiodysplasia: common in the elderly, painless, no warning, often large volume, fresh and clots mixed.

• Carcinoma of the caecum: more often causes anaemia than PR bleeding.

Colon

• Polyps/carcinoma: may be large volume or small, ?associated change in bowel habit, blood often mixed with stool.

• Diverticular disease: spontaneous onset, painless, large volume, mostly fresh blood, previous history of constipation.

• Ulcerative colitis: blood mixed with mucus, associated with systemic upset, long history, intermittent course, diarrhoea prominent.

• Ischaemic colitis: elderly, severe abdominal pain, AF, bloody diarrhoea, collapse and shock later.

Rectum

• Carcinoma of the rectum: change in bowel habit common, rarely large volumes.

• Proctitis: bloody mucus, purulent diarrhoea in infected, perianal irritation common.

• Solitary rectal ulcer: bleeding post-defaecation, small volumes, feeling of 'lump in anus', mucus discharge.

Anus

• Haemorrhoids: bright red bleeding post-defaecation, stops spontaneously, perianal irritation.

• Fissure *in ano*: extreme pain post-defaecation, small volumes bright red blood on stool and toilet paper.

• Carcinoma of the anus: elderly, mass in anus, small volumes bloody discharge, anal pain, unhealing ulcers.

• Perianal Crohn's disease.

17 Diarrhoea

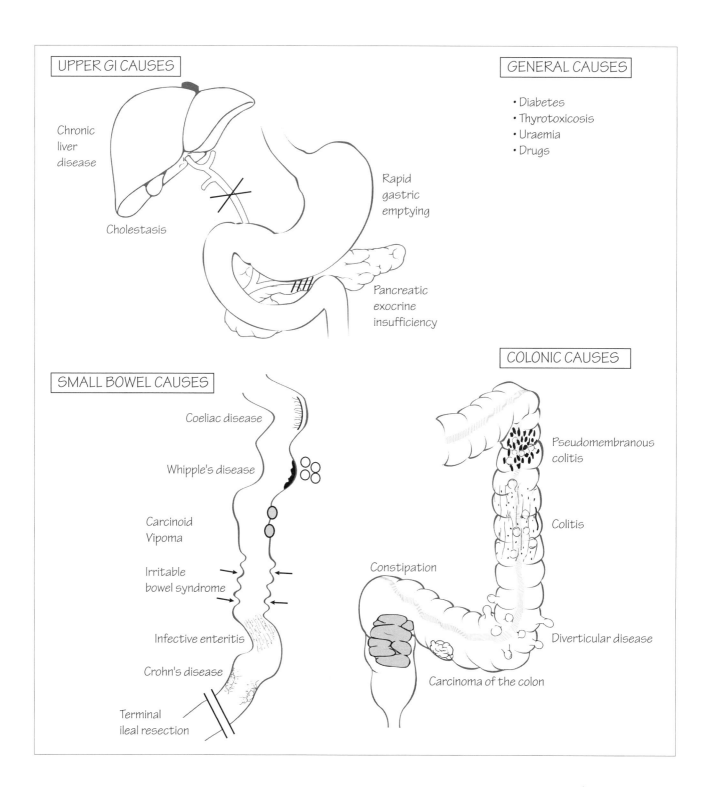

UPPER GI CAUSES

Chronic liver disease

Cholestasis

Rapid gastric emptying

Pancreatic exocrine insufficiency

GENERAL CAUSES

- Diabetes
- Thyrotoxicosis
- Uraemia
- Drugs

SMALL BOWEL CAUSES

Coeliac disease

Whipple's disease

Carcinoid Vipoma

Irritable bowel syndrome

Infective enteritis

Crohn's disease

Terminal ileal resection

COLONIC CAUSES

Pseudomembranous colitis

Colitis

Constipation

Diverticular disease

Carcinoma of the colon

Definition

Diarrhoea is defined as the passage of loose, liquid stool. *Urgency* is the sensation of the need to defaecate without being able to delay. It may indicate rectal irritability but also occurs where the volume of liquid stool is too large, causing the rectum to be overwhelmed as a storage vessel. *Frequency* merely reflects the number of stools passed and may or may not be associated with urgency or diarrhoea.

KEY POINTS

- Bloody diarrhoea is always pathological and usually indicates colitis of one form or another.
- Infective causes are common in acute transient diarrhoea.
- In diarrhoea of uncertain origin, remember the endocrine causes.
- Consider parasitic infections in a history of foreign travel.
- Alternating morning diarrhoea and normal/pelletty stools later in the day is rarely pathological.
- Diarrhoea developing in hospitalized patients may be due to *Clostridium difficile* infection—check for CD toxin in the stool.

Important diagnostic features

Acute diarrhoea

Infections

- *Shigella/Salmonella*: associated colicky abdominal pain, vomiting.
- Dysentery: blood and mucus in motions, ulcers in rectum and *Entamoeba histolytica* in the stool, fever, sweating, tachycardia.
- Cholera: severe diarrhoea, 'rice water' stool, dehydration, history of foreign travel.
- *Giardiasis*.

Antibiotics

Short-lived, self-limiting, mild colicky pain.

Pseudomembranous colitis

Caused by *Clostridium difficile* infection, characterized by severe diarrhoea which may be bloody but occasionally acute constipation may indicate severe disease. Characteristic features on colonoscopy.

Chronic diarrhoea

Small bowel disease

- Crohn's disease: diarrhoea, pain prominent, blood and mucus less common, young adults, long history, chronic malnourishment and weight loss.

- Coeliac disease: history of wheat and cereals intolerance, may present in adulthood with chronic diarrhoea and weight loss, abdominal pains.
- 'Blind loop' syndrome: frothy, foul-smelling liquid stool, due to bacterial overgrowth and fermentation, usually associated with previous surgery, may complicate Crohn's disease.

Large bowel disease

- Ulcerative colitis: intermittent, blood and mucus, colicky pains, young adults. May be a short history in first presentations. Rarely presents with acute fulminant colitis with acute abdominal signs.
- Colon cancer: older, occasional blood streaks and mucus, change in frequency may be the only feature, positive faecal occult blood, rectal mass.
- Irritable bowel syndrome: diarrhoea and constipation mixed, bloating, colicky pain, small stool pellets, never blood.
- Spurious: impacted faeces in rectum, liquefied stool passes around faecal obstruction, elderly, mental illness, constipating drugs.
- Polyps (villous) (rare): watery, mucoid diarrhoea, K^+ loss, commonest in rectum.
- Diverticular disease (rare).

Systemic disease

Thyrotoxicosis, anxiety, peptides from tumours (VIP, serotonin, substance P, calcitonin), laxative abuse.

KEY INVESTIGATIONS

- FBC: leucocytosis (infective causes, colitis), anaemia (colon cancer, ulcerative colitis, diverticular disease).
- Anti α-gliadin Abs: coeliac disease.
- Thyroid function tests: hyperthyroidism.
- Stool culture: infections (remember microscopy for parasites).
- Proctoscopy/sigmoidoscopy: cancer, colitis, polyps (simple, easy, cheap and safe; performed in outpatients).
- Flexible sigmoidoscopy: cancer, polyps, colitis, infections (relatively safe, well tolerated, high sensitivity).
- Colonoscopy: colitis (extent and severity), pseudomembranous colitis.
- Small bowel enema: Crohn's disease, coeliac disease, Whipple's disease.
- Faecal fat estimation/ERCP: pancreatic insufficiency.

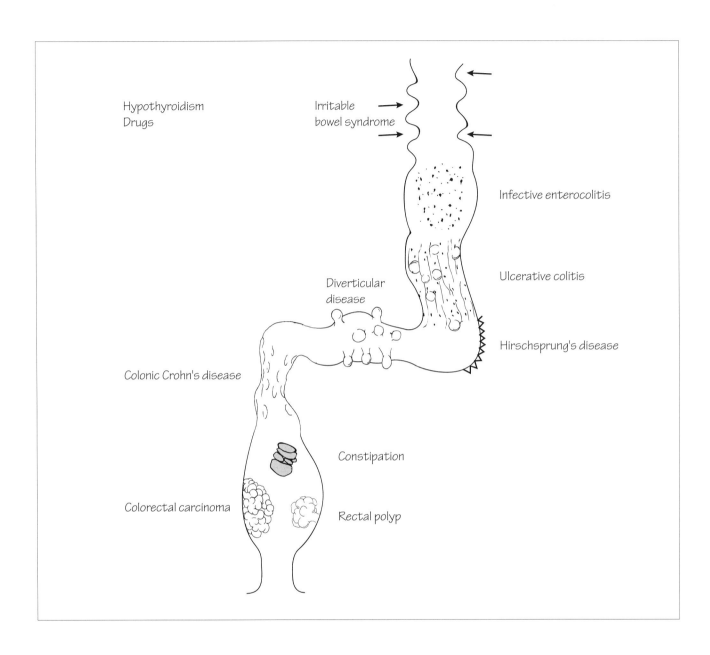

Hypothyroidism
Drugs

Irritable
bowel syndrome

Infective enterocolitis

Diverticular
disease

Ulcerative colitis

Hirschsprung's disease

Colonic Crohn's disease

Constipation

Colorectal carcinoma

Rectal polyp

Definitions

'*Normal*' *bowel habit* varies widely from person to person. Alterations in bowel habit are common manifestations of GI disease. *Constipation* is defined as infrequent or difficult evacuation of faeces and can be acute or chronic. *Absolute constipation* is defined as the inability to pass either faeces or flatus. *Diarrhoea* is an increase in the fluidity of stool.

> **KEY POINTS**
> • Acute constipation often indicates intestinal obstruction. The cardinal symptoms of obstruction are colicky abdominal pain, vomiting, constipation and distension.
> • Chronic constipation may be a lifelong problem or may develop slowly in later life.
> • All alterations in bowel habit that persist must be investigated for an underlying cause—colorectal neoplasms are common causes, especially in the elderly.

Important diagnostic features

Chronic constipation

Bowel disease

• Colon cancer: gradual onset, colicky abdominal pain, associated weight loss, anergia, anaemia, positive faecal occult bloods, abdominal mass.

• Diverticular disease: associated LIF pains, inflammatory episodes, rectal bleeding.

• Perianal pain, e.g. fissure, perianal abscess—due to spasm of the internal anal sphincter, common in children.

Adynamic bowel

• Hirschsprung's disease: constipation from birth, gross abdominal distension. Short-segment Hirschprung's disease (involving only the lower rectum) may present in adulthood with worsening chronic constipation and megarectum/megasigmoid.

• Drugs: opiates, anticholinergics, antipsychotics, secondary to chronic laxative abuse.

• Pregnancy: due to progesterone effects on smooth muscle of bowel wall.

> **KEY INVESTIGATIONS**
> • Rectal examination: rectal cancer, rectal adenoma.
> • FBC: anaemia from colon cancer, ulcerative colitis, diverticular disease.
> • Stool culture: infections (remember microscopy for parasites).
> • Proctoscopy/sigmoidoscopy: cancer, colitis, polyps (simple, easy, cheap and safe; performed in outpatients).
> • Flexible sigmoidoscopy: cancer, polyps, colitis, infections (relatively safe, well tolerated, high sensitivity).
> • Barium enema: best for tumours of proximal colon.
> • Colonoscopy: colitis (extent and severity).
> • Rectal biopsy (full thickness): Hirschsprung's disease.

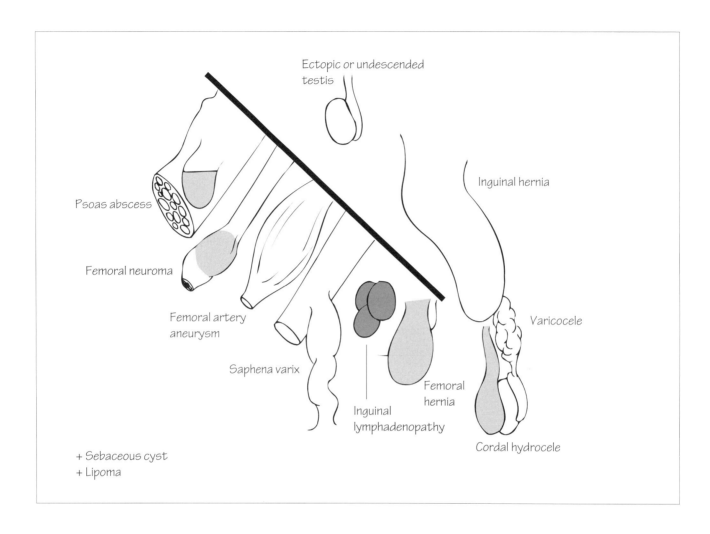

Ectopic or undescended testis

Inguinal hernia

Psoas abscess

Femoral neuroma

Femoral artery aneurysm

Saphena varix

Inguinal lymphadenopathy

Femoral hernia

Varicocele

Cordal hydrocele

+ Sebaceous cyst
+ Lipoma

Definition

Any swelling in the inguinal area or upper medial thigh.

> **KEY POINTS**
> • The groin crease does not mark the inguinal ligament in most people and is an unreliable landmark.
> • Inguinal hernias are common, always start above and medial to the pubic tubercle, may be medial or lateral to it and usually emphasize the groin crease on that side.
> • Femoral hernias always start below and lateral to the pubic tubercle and usually flatten the skin crease on that side.
> • Femoral hernias are commoner in women, are high risk and need urgent attention.
> • Masses in the groin and scrotum together are inguinal hernias.
> • Inguinal lymphadenopathy may be isolated or may be part of systemic lymphadenopathy. A cause should always be sought.

Important diagnostic features

The types, causes and features are listed below.

Inguinal

• Direct inguinal hernia: not controlled by pressure over internal ring, characteristically causes a 'forward' bulge in the groin, does not descend into the scrotum.
• Indirect inguinal hernia: controlled by pressure over internal ring, 'slides' through the inguinal canal, often descends into the scrotum.
• Undescended testis: often mass at the external ring or inguinal canal, associated with hypoplastic hemi-scrotum, frequently associated with indirect inguinal hernia.

• Spermatic cord: 'cordal' hydrocele, does not have a cough impulse, may be possible to define upper edge, fluctuates and transilluminates.
• Lipoma: soft, fleshy, does not transilluminate or fluctuate.

Femoral

• Femoral hernia: elderly women (mostly), may be tender and non-expansile, not reducible, groin crease often lost, high risk of strangulation and obstruction.
• Saphena varix: expansile, cough impulse, thrill on percussion of distal saphenous vein.
• Lymphadenopathy: hard, discrete nodules, often multiple or an indistinct mass.
• Femoral artery aneurysm: expansile, pulsatile, thrill and bruit may be present.
• Psoas abscess (rare): soft, fluctuant and compressible, lateral to the femoral artery, may be 'cold' abscesses caused by TB.
• Femoral neuroma (very rare): hard, smooth, moves laterally but not vertically, pressure may cause pain in the distribution of the femoral nerve.
• Hydrocele of femoral sac (very rare).

> **KEY INVESTIGATIONS**
> • FBC: causes of lymphadenopathy.
> • Ultrasound: femoral aneurysm, saphena varix, psoas abscess, ectopic testicle. Also sometimes useful to identify small femoral hernias.
> • CT scan: cause of psoas abscess.
> • Herniography: rarely needed to confirm presence of hernia if operative indication not clear.

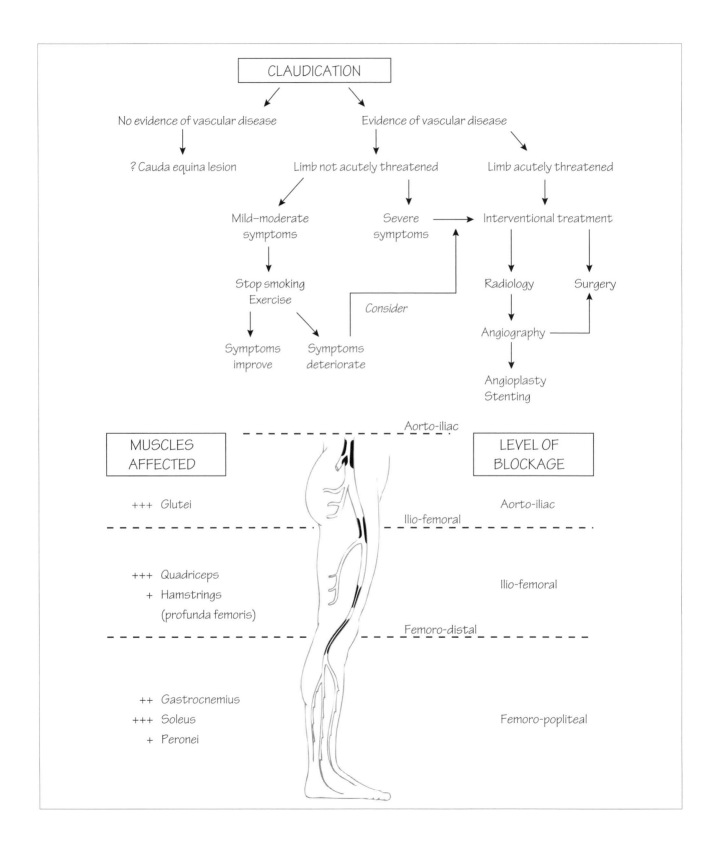

CLAUDICATION

No evidence of vascular disease   Evidence of vascular disease

? Cauda equina lesion   Limb not acutely threatened   Limb acutely threatened

Mild–moderate symptoms   Severe symptoms → Interventional treatment

Stop smoking Exercise

Consider

Radiology   Surgery

Symptoms improve   Symptoms deteriorate

Angiography

Angioplasty Stenting

Aorto-iliac

| MUSCLES AFFECTED | | LEVEL OF BLOCKAGE |

+++ Glutei   Aorto-iliac

Ilio-femoral

+++ Quadriceps
+ Hamstrings
(profunda femoris)

Ilio-femoral

Femoro-distal

++ Gastrocnemius
+++ Soleus
+ Peronei

Femoro-popliteal

Definition

Intermittent claudication is defined as an aching pain in the leg muscles, usually the calf, which is precipitated by walking and is relieved by rest.

Differential diagnosis

Vascular

Atheroma

• Typical patient: male, over 45 years, ischaemic heart disease, smoker, diabetic, overweight.

• Aortic occlusion: buttock, thigh and possibly calf claudication, impotence in males, absent femoral pulses and below in both legs (Leriche's syndrome).

• Iliac or common femoral stenosis: thigh and calf claudication, absent/weak femoral pulses in affected limb.

• Femoro-popliteal stenosis: calf claudication only, absent popliteal and distal pulses.

Neurological

Cauda equina

Elderly patients, history of chronic back pain, pain is bilateral and in the distribution of the S1–S3 dermatomes, may be accompanied by paraesthesia in the feet and loss of ankle jerks, all peripheral pulses palpable and legs well perfused.

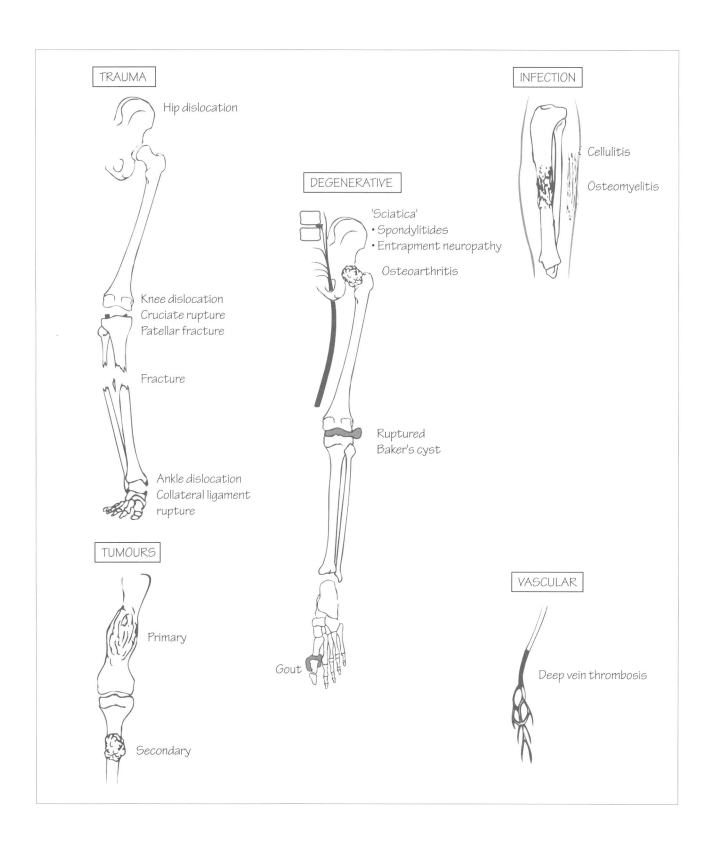

TRAUMA

Hip dislocation

Knee dislocation
Cruciate rupture
Patellar fracture

Fracture

Ankle dislocation
Collateral ligament
rupture

DEGENERATIVE

'Sciatica'
• Spondylitides
• Entrapment neuropathy

Osteoarthritis

Ruptured
Baker's cyst

Gout

INFECTION

Cellulitis

Osteomyelitis

TUMOURS

Primary

Secondary

VASCULAR

Deep vein thrombosis

Definitions

Acute leg pain is a subjective, unpleasant sensation felt somewhere in the lower limb. *Referred pain* is the perception of pain in an area remote from the site of origin of the pain, e.g. leg pain from lumbar disc herniation, knee pain from hip pathology. *Cramps* are involuntary, painful contractions of voluntary muscles. *Sciatica* is a nerve pain caused by irritation of the sciatic nerve roots characterized by lumbosacral pain radiating down the back of the thigh, lateral side of the calf and into the foot.

KEY POINTS
- May be due to pathology arising in any of the tissues of the leg.
- Constant or lasting pain suggests local pathology.
- Transient or intermittent pain suggests referred pathology.
- Systemic symptoms or upset suggests inflammation.

Important diagnostic features

Infection

- Infection of skin (cellulitis): painful, swollen, red, hot leg, associated systemic features—pyrexia, rigors, anorexia, commonly caused by *Streptococcus pyogenes*.
- Acute osteomyelitis: staphylococcal infection, effects metaphyses, acute pain, tenderness and oedema over the end of a long bone, common in children, may be history of skin infection or trauma.

Trauma

- Muscle: swollen, tender and painful, pain worse on attempted movement of the affected muscle.
- Bone: painful, tender. Swelling, deformity, discoloration, bruising and crepitus suggest fracture.

- Joints: painful, limited movement, deformity if dislocated, locking and instability with knee injury.

Degenerative

- Gout: first MTP joint (big toe), males, associated signs of joint inflammation.
- Disc herniation (sciatica): pain in distribution of one or two nerve roots, sudden onset, back pain and stiffness, lumbar scoliosis due to muscle spasm.
- Ruptured Baker's cyst: pain mostly behind the knee, previous history of knee arthritis, calf may be hot and swollen.

Tumours

Bone: deep pain, worse in morning and after exercise, overlying muscle tenderness, pathological fractures, primary (e.g. osteosarcoma, osteoclastoma) or secondary (e.g. breast, prostate, lung metastasis).

Vascular

DVT: calf pain, swelling, redness, prominent superficial veins, tender on calf compression, low-grade pyrexia.

KEY INVESTIGATIONS
- FBC: WCC in infection.
- D-Dimers: suspected DVT.
- Blood cultures: spreading cellulitis.
- Clotting: DVT.
- Plain X-ray: trauma, osteomyelitis, bone tumours, gout.
- MRI: suspected disc herniation.
- Duplex ultrasound: DVT.
- Venography: DVT where duplex not available or precise extent needed.

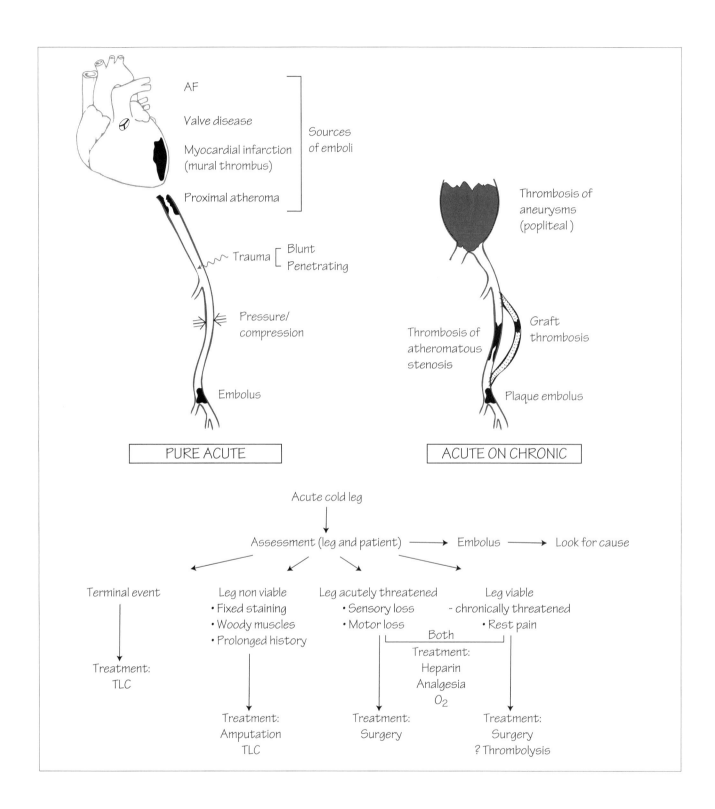

AF

Valve disease

Myocardial infarction
(mural thrombus)

Proximal atheroma

Sources
of emboli

Trauma [Blunt
Penetrating

Pressure/
compression

Embolus

PURE ACUTE

Thrombosis of
aneurysms
(popliteal)

Thrombosis of
atheromatous
stenosis

Graft
thrombosis

Plaque embolus

ACUTE ON CHRONIC

Acute cold leg

Assessment (leg and patient) → Embolus → Look for cause

Terminal event

Treatment:
TLC

Leg non viable
• Fixed staining
• Woody muscles
• Prolonged history

Treatment:
Amputation
TLC

Leg acutely threatened
• Sensory loss
• Motor loss

Leg viable
- chronically threatened
• Rest pain

Both
Treatment:
Heparin
Analgesia
O_2

Treatment:
Surgery

Treatment:
Surgery
? Thrombolysis

Definitions

The '*acute cold leg*' is a clinical syndrome of the sudden onset of symptoms indicative of the presence of ischaemia sufficient to threaten the viability of the limb or part of it.

> **KEY POINTS**
> - Remember the '6 Ps' of acute ischaemia—painful, pale, paraesthetic, paralysed, pulseless, perishingly cold.
> - All acute cold legs are a surgical emergency and require a prompt diagnosis.
> - 80% of acute cold legs presenting as an emergency have underlying chronic vascular pathology.
> - Fasciotomies should always be considered as part of treatment if a leg is being revascularized.

Important diagnostic features

Isolated arterial embolus

- Sudden-onset, severe ischaemia, no previous symptoms of vascular disease, previous history of atrial fibrillation/recent myocardial infarction, all peripheral pulses on the unaffected limb normal (suggesting no underlying peripheral vascular disease [PVD]).
- Limb usually acutely threatened due to complete occlusion with no collateral supply.
- Common sites of impaction are: popliteal bi(tri)furcation, distal superficial femoral artery (adductor canal), origin of the profunda femoris. 'Saddle' embolus at aortic bifurcation causes bilateral acute ischaemic limbs.

Trauma

- May be due to direct injury to the vessel or by secondary compression due to bone fragments or haematoma.
- Direct injuries may be due to: complete division of the vessel, distraction injury, damage and *in situ* thrombosis, foreign body, false aneurysm.

Thrombosis (*in situ*)

- Usually associated with underlying atheroma predisposing to thrombosis after minor trauma or immobility (after a fall or illness).
- May be subacute in onset, previous history of known vascular disease or intermittent claudication, associated risk factors for peripheral vascular disease, abnormal pulses in the unaffected limb.
- Paradoxically, the limb may not be as acutely threatened as in isolated arterial embolus since collateral vessels may already be present due to underlying disease.

Graft thrombosis

Often subacute in onset, limb not acutely threatened, progressive symptoms, loss of graft pulsation

Aneurysm thrombosis

- Commonest site—popliteal aneurysms.
- Sudden-onset limb ischaemia, acutely threatened, may be associated embolization as well, non-pulsatile mass in popliteal fossa, many have contralateral asymptomatic popliteal aneurysm.

> **KEY INVESTIGATIONS**
> - FBC: polycythaemia.
> - U+E: renal impairment, myonecrosis.
> - Clotting: thrombophilia.
> - ECG: atrial fibrillation, myocardial infarction, valve disease.
> - Duplex scanning: graft patency, popliteal aneurysm
> - Angiography: wherever possible—arterial embolism, thrombosis, underlying PVD.

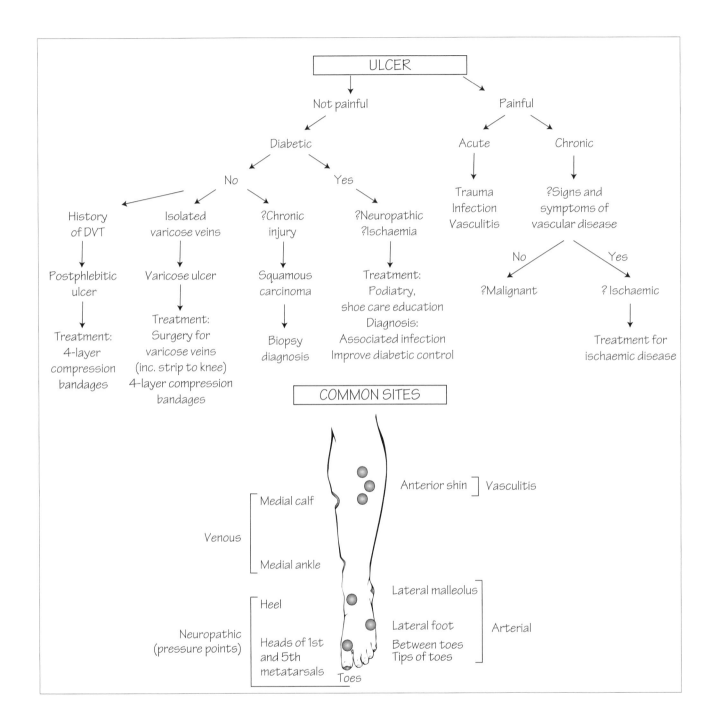

Definition

An *ulcer* is defined as an area of discontinuity of the surface epithelium.

KEY POINTS

- Pain suggests ischaemia or infection.
- Neuropathic ulcers occur over points of pressure and trauma.
- Marked worsening of a chronic ulcer suggests malignant change.
- The underlying cause must be treated first or the ulcer will not heal.
- Several precipitating causes may coexist (e.g. diabetes, PVD and neuropathy).
- Underlying varicose veins must be treated for venous ulcers.

Important diagnostic features

Venous ulcers

- Venous hypertension secondary to DVT or varicose veins: ulceration on the medial side of the leg, above the ankle, any size, shallow with sloping edges, bleeds after minor trauma, weeps readily, associated dermatoliposclerosis.
- If deep venous disease is suspected duplex scanning of the veins or venography is indicated.

Arterial ulcers

Occlusive arterial disease: painful ulcers, do not bleed, non-healing, lateral ankle, heel, metatarsal heads, tips of the toes, associated features of ischaemia, e.g. claudication, absent pulses, pallor. Elderly patients may present with 'blue toe' syndrome.

Diabetic ulcers

- Ischaemic: same as arterial ulcers.
- Neuropathic: deep, painless ulcers, plantar aspect of foot or toes, associated with cellulitis and deep tissue abscesses, warm foot, pulses may be present.

Malignant ulcers

- Squamous cell carcinoma: may arise *de novo* or malignant change in a chronic ulcer or burn (Marjolin's ulcer). Large ulcer, heaped up, everted edges. Lymphadenopathy—highly suspicious.
- Basal cell carcinoma: uncommon on the leg, rolled edges, pearly white.
- Malignant melanoma: lower limb is a common site, consider malignant if increase in size or pigmentation, bleeding, itching or ulceration.

Miscellaneous ulcers

- Trauma: may be caused by minor trauma. Predisposing factors are poor circulation, malnutrition or steroid treatment.
- Vasculitis (rare), e.g. rheumatoid arthritis, SLE.
- Infections (rare): syphilis, TB, tropical infections.
- Pyoderma gangrenosum: multiple necrotic ulcers over the legs that start as nodules. Seen with ulcerative colitis and Crohn's disease.

KEY INVESTIGATIONS

- FBC: infections.
- Glucose: diabetes.
- Special blood tests: TPHA (syphilis), ANCA (SLE), Rh factor.
- Ankle–brachial pressure index (ABI) measurement to exclude underlying PVD.
- Doppler ultrasound: assessment of venous disease, assessment of arterial disease (above the knee). Simple, cheap, highly sensitive, good screening test.
- Biopsy: malignancy. Melanoma—always excision biopsy. Others may be incision/'punch'.
- Venography/angiography: extent and severity of disease. Planning treatment.

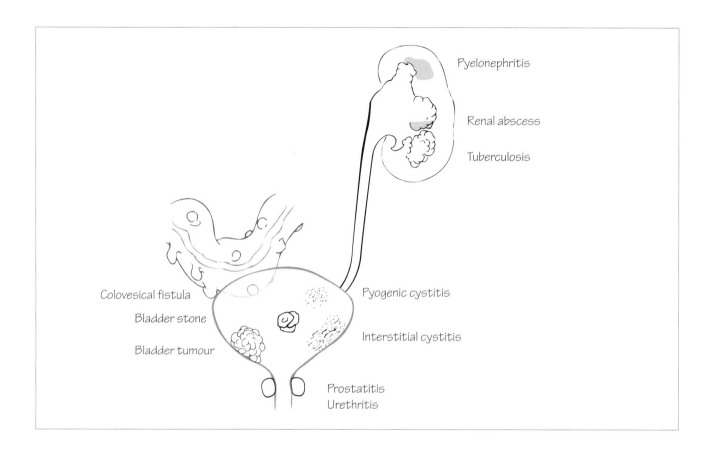

Definitions

Dysuria is defined as a pain that arises from an irritation of the urethra and is felt during micturition. *Frequency* indicates increased passage of urine during the daytime, while *nocturia* indicates increased passage of urine during the night. *Urgency* is an uncontrollable desire to micturate and may be associated with incontinence.

KEY POINTS
- UTI is the commonest cause of dysuria in adults.
- Systemic upset and loin pain suggest an ascending UTI (pyelonephritis).
- Elderly men with recurrent UTIs often have an underlying problem of bladder emptying due to prostate disease.
- Recurrent infections require investigation to exclude an underlying cause.
- Pneumaturia, 'bits' in the urine and coliform infections suggest a colovesical fistula.

Important diagnostic features
Urinary tract infection
Acute pyelonephritis
Cause: Upper tract infection.

Predisposing causes are:
- Outflow tract obstruction.
- Vesicoureteric reflux.
- Renal or bladder calculi.
- Diabetes mellitus.
- Neuropathic bladder dysfunction.

Features: Pyrexia, rigors, flank pain, dysuria, malaise, anorexia, leucocytosis, pyuria, bacteriuria, microscopic haematuria, C&S >100 000 organisms per ml.

Acute cystitis
Causes are:
- Lower tract infection.
- Usually coliform bacteria.
- Because of short urethra commoner in females.
- Proteus infections may indicate stone disease.

Features: Dysuria, frequency, urgency, suprapubic pain, low back pain, incontinence and microscopic haematuria.

Urethritis
Causes are:
- Sexually transmitted diseases.
- May be gonococcal, chlamydial or mycoplasmal.

Features: Dysuria and meatal pruritus, occurs 3–10 days after sexual contact, yellowish purulent urethral discharge suggests *Gonococcus*, thin mucoid discharge suggests *Chlamydia*.

Other causes of dysuria
Urethral syndrome
A condition characterized by frequency, urgency and dysuria in women with urine cultures showing no growth or low bacterial counts.

Vaginitis
Condition characterized by dysuria, pruritus and vaginal discharge. Urine cultures are negative, but vaginal cultures often reveal *Trichomonas vaginalis*, *Candida albicans* or *Haemophilus vaginalis*.

Bladder tumours
- Uncommon cause of dysuria, haematuria, sterile pyuria (no growth on MSU).
- Ultrasound: possible pyelonephritis/renal abscess, may show predisposing structural abnormality.
- DMSA scan: assesses renal function where renal damage suspected from recurrent sepsis.

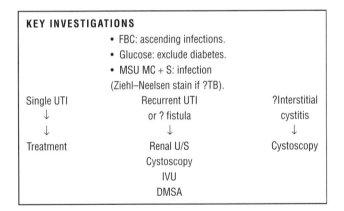

KEY INVESTIGATIONS
- FBC: ascending infections.
- Glucose: exclude diabetes.
- MSU MC + S: infection (Ziehl–Neelsen stain if ?TB).

Single UTI	Recurrent UTI or ? fistula	?Interstitial cystitis
↓	↓	↓
↓	↓	Cystoscopy
Treatment	Renal U/S Cystoscopy IVU DMSA	

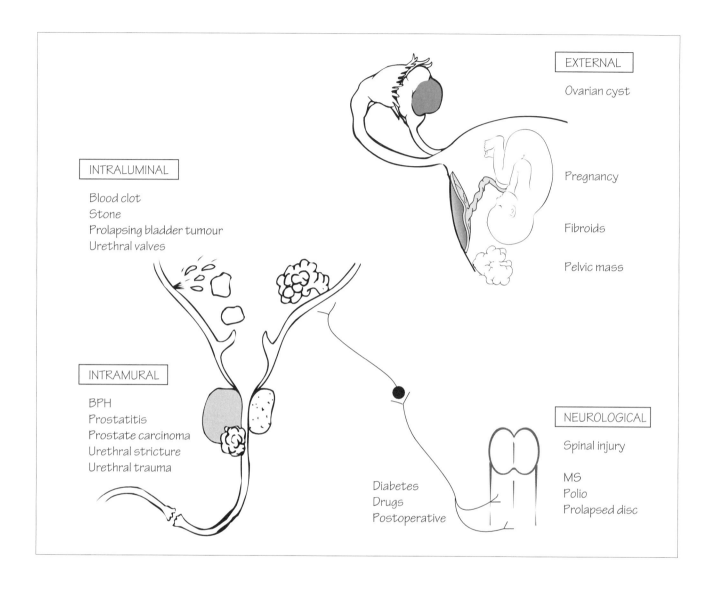

INTRALUMINAL

Blood clot
Stone
Prolapsing bladder tumour
Urethral valves

INTRAMURAL

BPH
Prostatitis
Prostate carcinoma
Urethral stricture
Urethral trauma

EXTERNAL

Ovarian cyst

Pregnancy

Fibroids

Pelvic mass

NEUROLOGICAL

Spinal injury

MS
Polio
Prolapsed disc

Diabetes
Drugs
Postoperative

Definitions

Urinary retention is defined as an inability to micturate. *Acute urinary retention* is the sudden inability to micturate in the presence of a painful bladder. *Chronic urinary retention* is the presence of an enlarged, full, painless bladder with or without difficulty in micturition. *Overflow incontinence* is an uncontrollable leakage and dribbling of urine from the urethra in the presence of a full bladder.

KEY POINTS

• **Acute retention** is characterized by pain, sensation of bladder fullness and a mildly distended bladder.
• Remember common causes:
  children—abdominal pain, drugs
  young—postoperative, drugs, acute UTI, trauma, haematuria
  elderly—acute on chronic retention with BPH, tumours, postoperative.
• **Chronic retention** is characterized by symptoms of bladder irritation (frequency, dysuria, small volume), or painless, marked distension, overflow incontinence (often associated with secondary UTI).
• Remember common causes:
  children—congenital abnormalities
  young—trauma, postoperative
  elderly—BPH, strictures, prostatic carcinoma.
• **Neurogenic retention**.
• Upper motor neurone causes produce chronic retention with reflex incontinence.
• Lower motor neurone causes produce chronic retention with overflow incontinence.
• Urinary retention is uncommon in young adults and almost always requires investigation to exclude underlying cause.
• Retention is common in elderly men—often due to prostate pathology.

Differential diagnosis
Mechanical

In the lumen of the urethra
• Congenital valves (rare): neonates, males, recurrent UTIs.
• Foreign body (rare).

• Stones (rare): acute pain in penis and glans.
• Tumour (rare): TCC or squamous cell carcinoma, history of haematuria, working in dye or rubber industry.

In the wall of the urethra
• BPH: frequency, nocturia, hesitancy, poor stream, dribbling, urgency.
• Tumour: as above.
• Stricture: history of trauma or serious infection, gradual onset of poor stream.
• Trauma: blood at meatus.

Outside the wall of the urethra
• Pregnancy.
• Fibroids: palpable, bulky uterus, menorrhagia, dysmenorrhoea.
• Ovarian cyst: mobile iliac fossa mass.
• Faecal impaction: spurious diarrhoea.

Neurological
• Postoperative: pain, drugs, pelvic nerve disturbance.
• Spinal cord injuries: acute phase is lower motor neurone type, late phase is upper motor neurone type.
• Drugs: narcotics, anticholinergics, antihistamines, antipsychotics.
• Diabetes: progressive lower motor neurone pattern.
• Idiopathic: detrusor sphincter dyssynergia, ?bladder neurone degeneration.

KEY INVESTIGATIONS

• U+E: renal function.
• MSU MC+S: associated infection, include cytology where tumour suspected.
• Cystography: urethral valves, strictures.
• IVU: renal/bladder stones.
• Urodynamics: allows identification and assessment of neurological problems, assesses BPH.
• Cystoscopy.

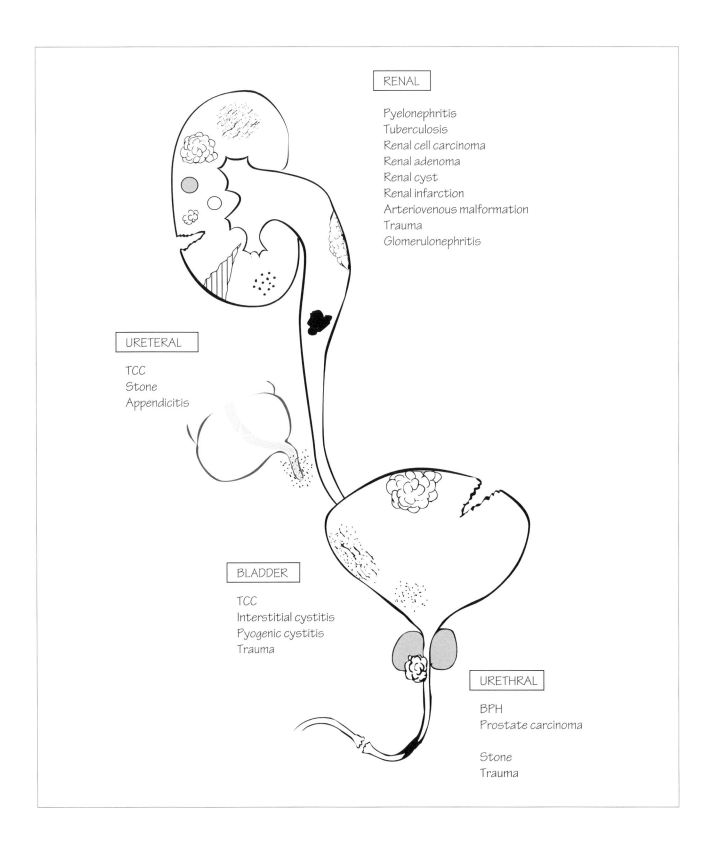

RENAL

Pyelonephritis
Tuberculosis
Renal cell carcinoma
Renal adenoma
Renal cyst
Renal infarction
Arteriovenous malformation
Trauma
Glomerulonephritis

URETERAL

TCC
Stone
Appendicitis

BLADDER

TCC
Interstitial cystitis
Pyogenic cystitis
Trauma

URETHRAL

BPH
Prostate carcinoma

Stone
Trauma

Definitions

Haematuria is the passage of blood in the urine. *Frank haematuria* is the presence of blood on macroscopic examination, while *microscopic haematuria* indicates that RBCs are only seen on microscopy. *Haemoglobinuria* is defined as the presence of free Hb in the urine.

KEY POINTS

• Haematuria always requires investigation to exclude an underlying cause.

• Initial haematuria (blood on commencing urination) suggests a urethral cause.

• Terminal haematuria (blood after passing urine) suggests a bladder base or prostatic cause.

• Ribbon clots suggest a pelvi-ureteric cause.

• Renal bleeding can mimic colic due to clots passing down the ureter.

Important diagnostic features

Kidney

• Trauma: mild to moderate trauma commonly causes renal bleeding, severe injuries may not bleed (avulsed kidney—complete disruption).

• Tumours: may be profuse or intermittent.

• Renal cell carcinoma: associated mass, loin pain, clot colic or fever, occasional polycythaemia, hypercalcaemia and hypertension.

• TCC: characteristically painless, intermittent haematuria.

• Calculus: severe loin/groin pain, gross or microscopic, associated infection.

• Glomerulonephritis: usually microscopic, associated systemic disease (e.g. SLE).

• Pyelonephritis (rare).

• Renal tuberculosis (rare): sterile pyuria, weight loss, anorexia, PUO, increased frequency of micturition day and night.

• Polycystic disease (rare): palpable kidneys, hypertension, chronic renal failure.

• Renal arteriovenous malformation or simple cyst (very rare): painless, no other symptoms.

• Renal infarction (very rare): may be caused by an arterial embolus, painful tender kidney.

Ureter

• Calculus: severe loin/groin pain, gross or microscopic, associated infection.

• TCC: see below.

Bladder

• Calculus: sudden cessation of micturition, pain in perineum and tip of penis.

• TCC: characteristically painless, intermittent haematuria, history of work in rubber or dye industries.

• Acute cystitis: suprapubic pain, dysuria, frequency and bacteriuria.

• Interstitial cystitis (rare): may be autoimmune, drug or radiation induced, frequency and dysuria common.

• Schistosomiasis (very rare): history of foreign travel, especially North Africa.

Prostate

• BPH: painless haematuria, associated obstructive symptoms, recurrent UTI.

• Carcinoma (rare).

Urethra

• Trauma: blood at meatus, history of direct blow to perineum, acute retention.

• Calculus (rare).

• Urethritis (rare).

KEY INVESTIGATIONS

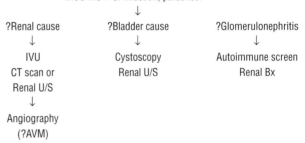

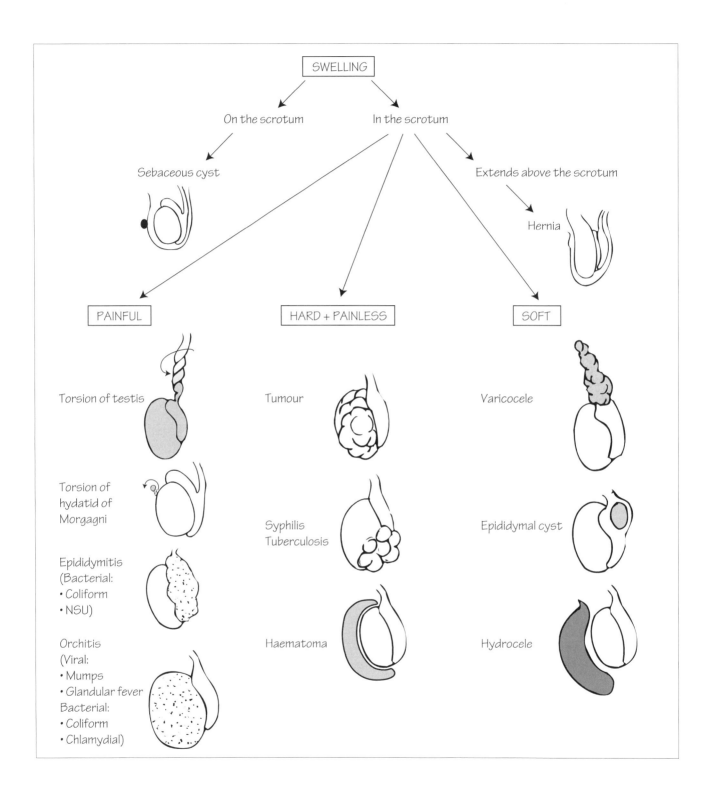

Definition

Any swelling in or on the scrotum or its contents.

Differential diagnosis

The causes and features are listed below.

Scrotum

• Sebaceous cyst: attached to the skin, just fluctuant, does not transilluminate.

• Infantile scrotal oedema: acute idiopathic scrotal swelling, hot, tender, bright red, testicle less tender than in torsion, commonest in young boys.

Testis

Painful conditions

• Orchitis: confined to testis, young men.

• Epididymo-orchitis: painful and swollen, epididymis more than testis, associated erythema of scrotum, fever and pyuria, unusual below the age of 25 years, pain relieved by elevating the testis.

• Torsion of the testis: rapid onset, pubertal males, often high investment of tunica vaginalis on the cord—'bellclapper testis', testis may lie high and transversely in the scrotum, 'knot' in the cord may be felt.

• Torsion of appendix testis: mimics full torsion, early signs are a lump at the upper pole of the testis and a blue spot on transillumination, later the whole testis becomes swollen, may require explorative surgery to exclude full torsion.

Hard conditions

• Testicular tumour: painless swelling, younger adult men (20–50 years), may have lax secondary hydrocele, associated abdominal lymphadenopathy.

• Haematocele: firm, does not transilluminate, testis cannot usually be felt, history of trauma.

• Syphilitic gummata—firm, rubbery, usually associated with other features of secondary syphilis. TB—uncommon outside developing world, usually associated with miliary disease.

Soft conditions

• Hydrocele: soft, fluctuant, transilluminates brilliantly, testis may be difficult to feel, new onset or rapidly recurrent hydrocele suggests an underlying testicular cause.

• Epididymal cyst: separate and behind the testis, transilluminates well, may be quite large.

• Varicocele: a collection of dilated and tortuous veins in the spermatic cord—'bag of worms' on examination, commoner on the left, associated with a dragging sensation, occasional haematospermia.

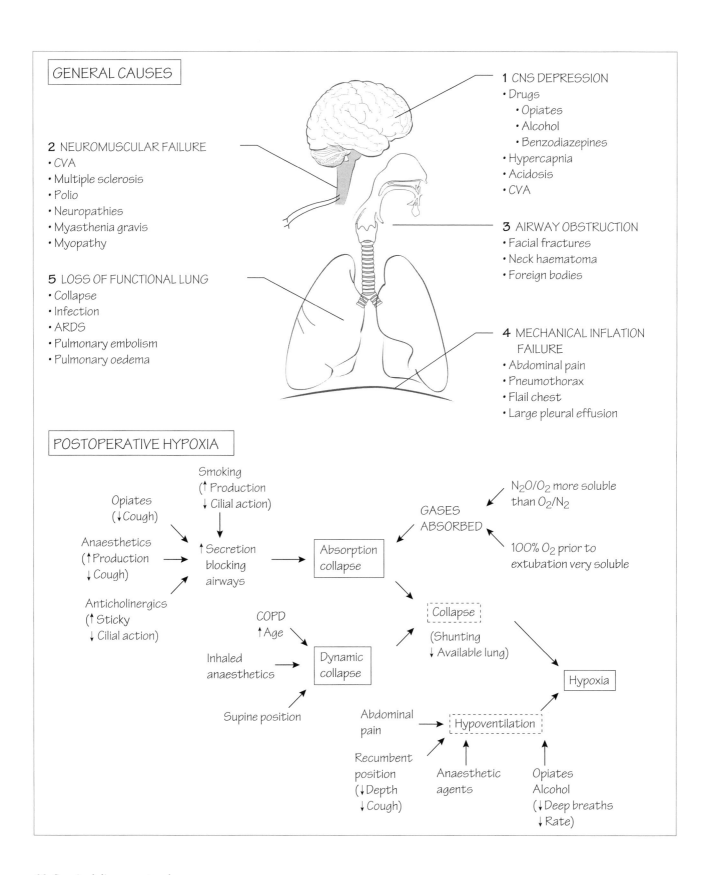

GENERAL CAUSES

1 CNS DEPRESSION
- Drugs
  - Opiates
  - Alcohol
  - Benzodiazepines
- Hypercapnia
- Acidosis
- CVA

2 NEUROMUSCULAR FAILURE
- CVA
- Multiple sclerosis
- Polio
- Neuropathies
- Myasthenia gravis
- Myopathy

3 AIRWAY OBSTRUCTION
- Facial fractures
- Neck haematoma
- Foreign bodies

5 LOSS OF FUNCTIONAL LUNG
- Collapse
- Infection
- ARDS
- Pulmonary embolism
- Pulmonary oedema

4 MECHANICAL INFLATION FAILURE
- Abdominal pain
- Pneumothorax
- Flail chest
- Large pleural effusion

POSTOPERATIVE HYPOXIA

Opiates ($\downarrow$ Cough)

Smoking ($\uparrow$ Production $\downarrow$ Cilial action)

Anaesthetics ($\uparrow$ Production $\downarrow$ Cough)

Anticholinergics ($\uparrow$ Sticky $\downarrow$ Cilial action)

$\uparrow$ Secretion blocking airways

Absorption collapse

GASES ABSORBED

N_2O/O_2 more soluble than O_2/N_2

100% O_2 prior to extubation very soluble

COPD $\uparrow$ Age

Inhaled anaesthetics

Dynamic collapse

Supine position

Collapse (Shunting $\downarrow$ Available lung)

Hypoxia

Abdominal pain

Recumbent position ($\downarrow$ Depth $\downarrow$ Cough)

Anaesthetic agents

Opiates Alcohol ($\downarrow$ Deep breaths $\downarrow$ Rate)

Hypoventilation

Definitions

Hypoxia is defined as a lack of O_2 (usually meaning lack of O_2 delivery to tissues or cells). *Hypoxaemia* is a lack of O_2 in arterial blood. *Apnoea* means cessation of breathing in expiration.

Common causes

Postoperative causes

- CNS depression, e.g. post-anaesthesia.
- Airway obstruction, e.g. aspiration of blood or vomit.
- Poor ventilation, e.g. abdominal pain, mechanical disruption to ventilation.
- Loss of functioning lung, e.g. ventilation–perfusion mismatch (pulmonary embolism, pneumothorax, collapse/consolidation).

General causes

- CNS depression, e.g. opiates, CVA, head injury.
- Airway obstruction, e.g. facial fractures, aspiration of blood or vomit, thyroid disease or cervical malignancy.
- Poor ventilation, e.g. pleural effusions, neuromuscular failure.
- Loss of functioning lung, e.g. ventilation–perfusion mismatch (pulmonary embolism, pneumothorax, collapse/consolidation), right to left pulmonary shunt.

KEY POINTS

- 80% of patients following upper abdominal surgery are hypoxic during the first 48 h postoperatively. Have a high index of suspicion and treat prophylactically.
- Adequate analgesia is more important than the sedative effects of opiates—ensure good analgesia in all postoperative patients.
- Ensure the dynamics of respiration are adequate—upright position, abdominal support, humidified O_2.
- Acutely confused (elderly) patients on a surgical ward are hypoxic until proven otherwise.
- Pulse oximetry saturations of less than 85% equate to an arterial Po_2 <8 kPa and are unreliable in patients with poor peripheral perfusion.

Analgesia in postoperative patients

- Opiates: powerful, highly effective if given by correct route (e.g. PCA) but antitussive, sedative only in overdose.

- Epidural: excellent for upper abdominal/thoracic surgery, can cause hypotension by relative hypovolaemia.

Clinical features

In the unconscious patient

- Central cyanosis.
- Abnormal respirations.
- Hypotension.

In the conscious patient

- Central cyanosis.
- Anxiety, restlessness and confusion.
- Tachypnoea.
- Tachycardia, dysrhythmias (AF) and hypotension.

Key investigations

- Pulse oximetry saturations: give a guide to arterial oxygenation.
- Arterial blood gases (Pco_2 Po_2 pH base excess): respiratory acidosis, metabolic acidosis later.
- Chest X-ray: ?collapse/pneumothorax/consolidation.
- ECG: AF.

ESSENTIAL MANAGEMENT

- **Airway** control.
- Triple airway manoeuvre, suction secretions, clear oropharynx.
- Consider endotracheal intubation in CNS depression/exhausted patients (rising Pco_2), neuromuscular failure.
- Consider surgical airway (cricothyroidotomy/mini-tracheostomy) in facial trauma, upper airway obstruction.
- **Breathing**.
- Position patient—upright.
- Adequate analgesia.
- Supplemental O_2—mask/bag/ventilation.
- Support respiratory physiology—physiotherapy, humidified gases, encouraging coughing, bronchodilators.
- **Circulatory** support.
- Maintain cardiac output.
- Ensure adequate fluid resuscitation.
- **Determine** and treat the cause.

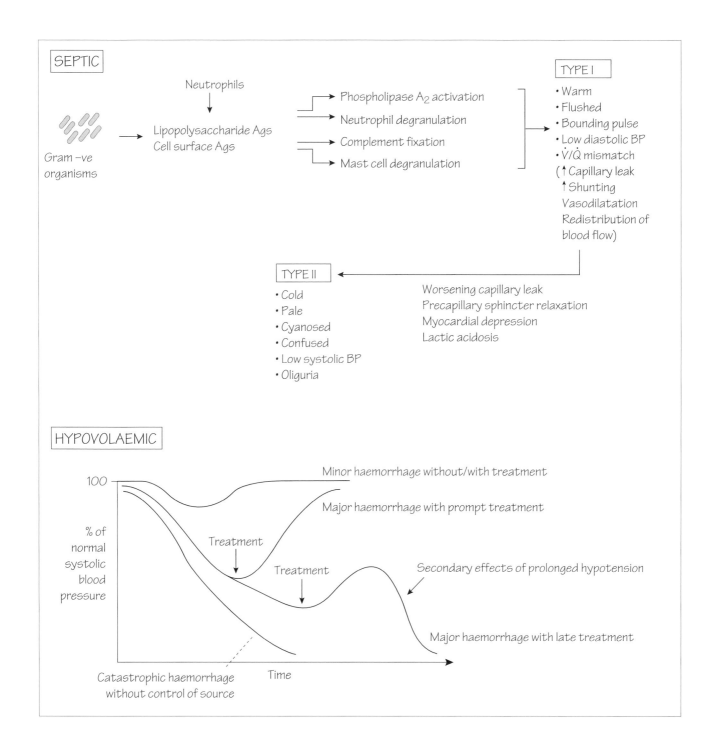

Definitions

Shock is defined as a state of acute inadequate or inappropriate tissue perfusion resulting in generalized cellular hypoxia and dysfunction.

> **KEY POINTS**
> - Identify the cause early and begin treatment quickly.
> - Shock in surgical patients is often overlooked—unwell, confused, restless patients may well be shocked.
> - Unless a cardiogenic cause is obvious, treat shock with urgent fluid resuscitation.
> - Worsening clinical status despite adequate volume replacement suggests the need for intensive care.

Common causes

Hypovolaemic

- Blood loss (ruptured abdominal aortic aneurysm, upper GI bleed, multiple fractures, etc.).
- Plasma loss (burns, pancreatitis).
- Extracellular fluid losses (vomiting, diarrhoea, intestinal fistula).

Cardiogenic

- Myocardial infarction.
- Dysrhythmias (AF, VT, AFlutter).
- Pulmonary embolus.
- Cardiac tamponade.
- Valvular heart disease

Septic

Gram –ve or, less often, Gram +ve infections.

Anaphylactic/distributive

Release of vasoactive substances when a sensitized individual is exposed to the appropriate antigen.

Clinical features

Hypovolaemic and cardiogenic

- Pallor, coldness, sweating and restlessness.
- Tachycardia, weak pulse, low BP and oliguria.

Septic

- Initially warm, flushed skin and bounding pulse.
- Later confusion and low output picture.

Investigations and assessment

- Monitor pulse, BP, temperature, respiratory rate and urinary output.
- Establish good i.v. access and set up CVP line (possibly Swan–Ganz catheter as well).
- ECG, cardiac enzymes, echocardiography.
- Hb, Hct, U+E, creatinine.
- Group and crossmatch blood: haemorrhage.
- Blood cultures: sepsis.
- Arterial blood gases.

Complications

- 'SIRS' (see p. 70) may ensue if shock not corrected.
- Acute renal failure (acute tubular necrosis).
- Hepatic failure.
- Stress ulceration.

ESSENTIAL MANAGEMENT

- **Airway and breathing**: give 100% O$_2$, sit up, consider ventilatory support if necessary.
- **Circulation**: ensure good IV access, urinary catheter, monitor cardiac rate and rhythm.

↓

Anaphylactic	Cardiogenic	Septic	Hypovolaemic
• i.v. fluids.	• Optimize rate and rhythm (e.g. cardioversion, drugs).	• Fluids to restore circulating volume.	• Identify and arrest losses (may include surgery).
• i.v. adrenaline.	• Optimize preload (e.g. adequate volume, diuretics).	• Antibiotics or surgery.	• Restore circulating volume (crystalloids, colloids or blood).
• i.v. antihistamines.	• Optimize afterload (e.g. vasoconstrictors/dilators).	• Support cardiac function (e.g. inotropes).	• Support cardiac function.
• i.v. hydrocortisone.	• Optimize cardiac function (e.g. thrombolytic therapy, inotropes, assist devices).		

Deal with the cause of the shock: e.g. stop the bleeding, drain the abscess, remove the source of the anaphylactic antigen, etc.

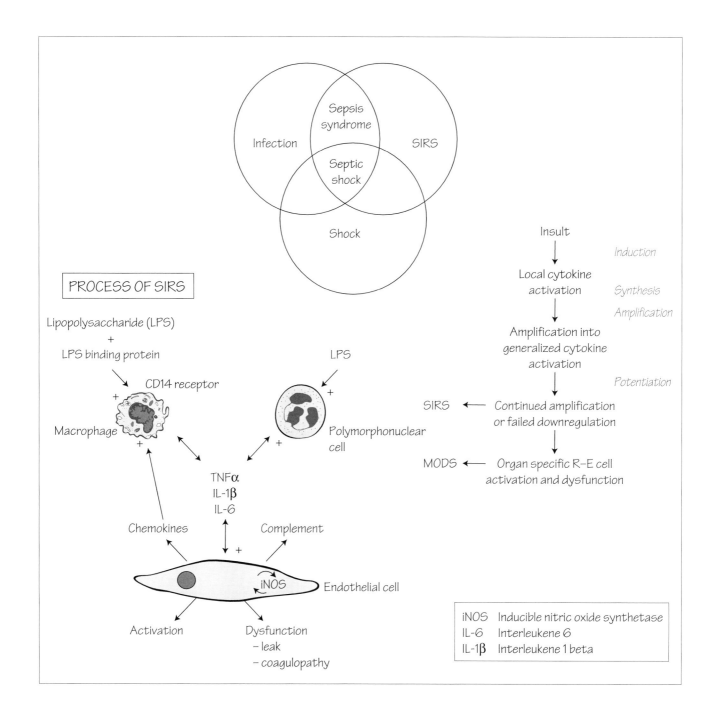

PROCESS OF SIRS

Lipopolysaccharide (LPS)
+
LPS binding protein

CD14 receptor

Macrophage

LPS

Polymorphonuclear cell

TNFα
IL-1β
IL-6

Chemokines

Complement

iNOS

Endothelial cell

Activation

Dysfunction
– leak
– coagulopathy

iNOS	Inducible nitric oxide synthetase
IL-6	Interleukene 6
IL-1β	Interleukene 1 beta

Insult — *Induction*

Local cytokine activation — *Synthesis*

Amplification

Amplification into generalized cytokine activation

Potentiation

SIRS ← Continued amplification or failed downregulation

MODS ← Organ specific R–E cell activation and dysfunction

Definitions

SIRS (systemic inflammatory response syndrome) is a systemic inflammatory response characterized by the presence of two or more of the following:

- hyperthermia $>38°C$ or hypothermia $<36°C$
- tachycardia >90 bpm
- tachypnoea >20 r.p.m. or $Pa_{CO_2} <4.3$ kPa
- neutrophilia $>12 \times 10^{-9}$ l^{-1} or neutropenia $<4 \times 10^{-9}$ l^{-1}.

Sepsis syndrome is a state of SIRS with proven infection. *Septic shock* is *sepsis* with systemic shock.

MODS (multiple organ dysfunction syndrome) is a state of derangement of physiology such that organ function cannot maintain homeostasis.

The common terminal pathways for organ damage and dysfunction are vasodilatation, capillary leak, intravascular coagulation and endothelial cell activation.

KEY POINTS

- SIRS is more common in surgical patients than is diagnosed.
- Early treatment of SIRS may reduce the risk of MODS developing.
- The role of treatment is to eliminate any causative factor and support the cardiovascular and respiratory physiology until the patient can recover.
- Overall mortality is 7% for a diagnosis of SIRS, 14% for sepsis syndrome and 40% for established septic shock.

Common surgical causes

- Acute pancreatitis.
- Perforated viscus with peritonitis.
- Fulminant colitis.
- Multiple trauma.
- Massive blood transfusion.
- Aspiration pneumonia.
- Ischaemia reperfusion injury.

Causation and treatments

TNFα

TNFα is both released by and activates macrophages and neutrophils. It is cytotoxic to endothelial cells and parenchymal cells of end organs. There is no clear evidence that anti-TNFα therapy is effective in SIRS.

Lipopolysaccharide (LPS)

Released from Gram $-$ve bacterial cell walls, activates macrophages via attachment of LPS binding protein and activation of CD14 molecules on the cell surface. There is no proven value for anti-LPS antibody treatment.

Interleukines

IL-6 and IL-1α cause endothelial cell activation and damage. They promote complement and chemokines release. High-dose intravenous steroids have little role in established SIRS (probably because of multiple pathways of activation). Steroids for early SIRS are unproven.

Platelet activating factor (PAF)

Implicated particularly in acute pancreatitis, no proven role for anti-PAF antibody treatment.

Inducible nitric oxide synthetase (iNOS)

Synthesized by activated endothelial cells, activates endothelial cells and leucocytes, potent negative ionotrope.

31 Acute renal failure

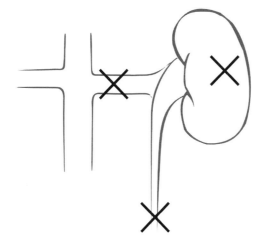

CAUSES

PRERENAL
Hypoperfusion
• Hypovolaemia
• Septicaemia
• Hypoxaemia
• Nephrotoxins
• Pancreatitis
• Liver cell dysfunction
　• Bilirubin
　• Other toxins

RENAL
• Any established cause
　of prerenal or postrenal
• Glomerular damage
　• Glomerulonephritis
• Tubular damage
　• Toxins
　• Drugs
　• Pyelonephritis
• Vascular damage
　• Acute vasculitis
　• Diabetes
　• Hypertension

POSTRENAL
• Primary tumours
• Secondary tumours — invasion
• Stones
• Blood clots
• Bladder obstruction
• Infestations (worms)

FEATURES

	Normal	Prerenal	Renal	Postrenal
$U_{osmolality}$	Approx 400–500 mosm/kg	> 500	<400	Normal
U_{Na^+}	10–20 mmol/l	< 10	> 20	Normal
U_{urea}/P_{urea}	Approx 5/1	> 10/1	3/1–1/1	Normal
U_{osm}/P_{osm}	Approx 1.5/1	> 2/1	< 1.1/1	Normal
Findings	—	Concentrated urine ? Findings due to cause	Casts RBCs Protein	Normal urine ? Findings due to cause

Definitions

Acute renal failure is a sudden deterioration in renal function such that neither kidney is capable of excreting body waste products (e.g. urea, creatinine, potassium) that accumulate in the blood. It is fatal unless treated. *Anuria* means no urine is passed. *Oliguria* means that less than 0.5 ml/kg/h is passed.

> **KEY POINTS**
> - Oliguria in a surgical patient is an emergency and the cause must be identified and treated promptly.
> - Prompt correction of pre-renal causes may prevent the development of established renal failure.
> - Ensure the oliguric patient is normovolaemic as far as possible before starting diuretics or other therapies.
> - Don't use blind, large fluid challenges, especially in the elderly—if necessary use a CVP line.
> - Established renal failure requires specialist support as electrolyte and fluid imbalances can be rapid in onset and difficult to manage.

Common causes

Pre-renal failure
- Shock causing reduced renal perfusion.
- Pancreatitis.

Intrinsic renal failure
- Shock causing renal ischaemia (ATN).
- Nephrotoxins (aminoglycosides, myoglobin).
- Acute glomerulonephritis.
- Severe pyelonephritis.
- Hypertension and diabetes mellitus.

Post-renal failure
- Urinary tract obstruction, e.g. prostatic hypertrophy.
- Obstructing renal calculi.

Clinical features

Specific to the cause
Hypovolaemia: cool peripheries, tachycardia, confusion, restlessness, dry mucous membranes.

Oliguric phase
(May last hours/days/weeks)
- Oliguria.
- Uraemia: dyspnoea, confusion, drowsiness, coma.
- Nausea, vomiting, hiccoughs, diarrhoea.
- Anaemia, coagulopathy, GI haemorrhage.

- Fluid retention: hypervolaemia, hypertension.
- Hyperkalaemia: dysrrhythmias.
- Acidosis.

Polyuric (recovery) phase
(May last days/weeks)
- Polyuria: hypovolaemia, hypotension.
- Hyponatraemia.
- Hypokalaemia.

Investigations
- Urinalysis (see opposite page).
- U+E (especially K^+).
- Creatinine estimation.
- ECG/chest X-ray.
- Arterial blood gases: metabolic acidosis (N Po_2, Lo Pco_2, Lo pH, Hi base deficit).

ESSENTIAL MANAGEMENT

Prevention
- Keep at-risk patients (e.g. patients with obstructive jaundice) well hydrated pre- and perioperatively.
- Protect renal function in selected patients with drugs such as dopamine and mannitol.
- Monitor renal function regularly in patients on nephrotoxic drugs (e.g. gentamicin).

Identification
- Exclude urinary retention as a cause of anuria by catheterization.
- Correct hypovolaemia as far as possible. Use appropriate fluid boluses—if necessary guided by a CVP monitor.
- A trial of bolus high-dose loop diuretics may be appropriate in a normovolaemic patient.
- Dopamine infusions may be necessary but suggest the need for HDU or ICU care.

Treatment of established renal failure
- Maintain fluid and electrolyte balance.
- Water intake 400 ml/day + measured losses.
- Na^+ intake limited to replace loss only.
- K^+ intake nil (dextrose and insulin and/or ion-exchange resins are required to control hyperkalaemia).
- Diet: high calorie, low protein in a small volume of fluid.
- Acidosis: sodium bicarbonate.
- Treat any infection.
- Dialysis: peritoneal, ultrafiltration, haemodialysis (usually indicated for hypervolaemia, hyperkalaemia or acidosis).

---

32 Fractures

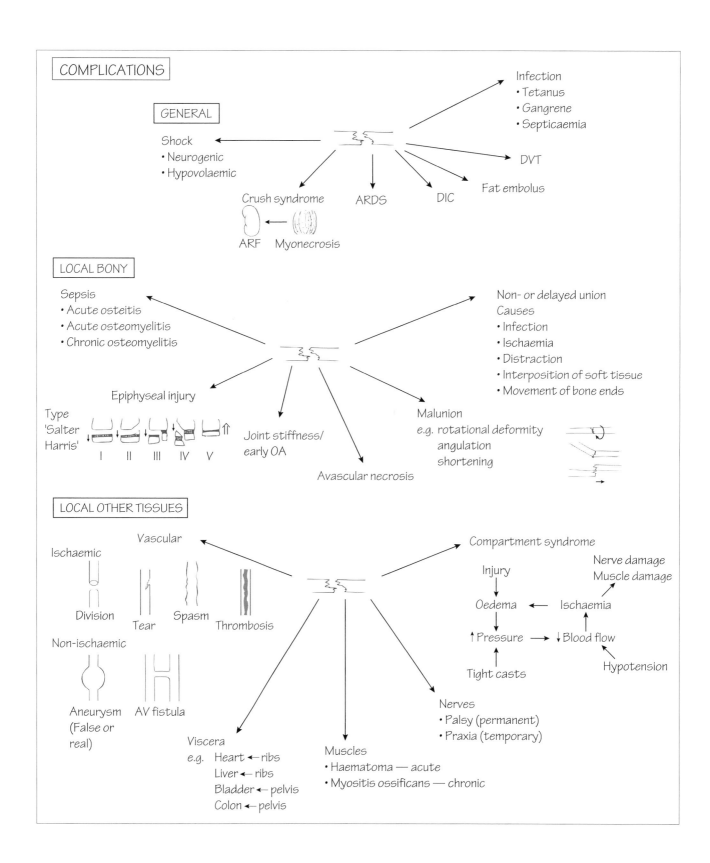

COMPLICATIONS

GENERAL

Infection
• Tetanus
• Gangrene
• Septicaemia

Shock
• Neurogenic
• Hypovolaemic

DVT

Crush syndrome

ARDS   DIC   Fat embolus

ARF   Myonecrosis

LOCAL BONY

Sepsis
• Acute osteitis
• Acute osteomyelitis
• Chronic osteomyelitis

Non- or delayed union
Causes
• Infection
• Ischaemia
• Distraction
• Interposition of soft tissue
• Movement of bone ends

Epiphyseal injury

Type
'Salter
Harris'
I   II   III   IV   V

Joint stiffness/
early OA

Malunion
e.g. rotational deformity
        angulation
        shortening

Avascular necrosis

LOCAL OTHER TISSUES

Vascular

Ischaemic

Division
Tear   Spasm   Thrombosis

Non-ischaemic

Aneurysm
(False or
real)

AV fistula

Viscera
e.g. Heart ← ribs
       Liver ← ribs
       Bladder ← pelvis
       Colon ← pelvis

Muscles
• Haematoma — acute
• Myositis ossificans — chronic

Compartment syndrome

Nerve damage
Muscle damage

Injury

Oedema ← Ischaemia

↑Pressure → ↓Blood flow

Tight casts   Hypotension

Nerves
• Palsy (permanent)
• Praxia (temporary)

Definitions

- A *fracture* is a break in the continuity of a bone.
- Fractures may be *transverse*, *oblique* or *spiral* in shape.
- In a *greenstick* fracture, only one side of the bone is fractured, the other simply bends (usually immature bones).
- A *comminuted* fracture is one in which there are more than two fragments of bone.
- In a *complicated* fracture, some other structure is also damaged (e.g. a nerve or blood vessel).
- In a *compound* fracture, there is a break in the overlying skin (or nearby viscera) with potential contamination of the bone ends.
- A *pathological* fracture is one through a bone weakened by disease, e.g. a metastasis.

KEY POINTS
- Always consider multiple injury in patients presenting with fractures.
- Compound fractures are a surgical emergency and require appropriate measures to prevent infection, including tetanus prevention.
- Always image the joints above and below a long bone fracture.

Common causes

Fractures occur when excessive force is applied to a normal bone or moderate force to a diseased bone, e.g. osteoporosis.

Clinical features

- Pain.
- Loss of function.
- Deformity, tenderness and swelling.
- Discoloration or bruising.
- (Crepitus, not to be elicited!)

Investigations

- Radiographs in two planes (look for lucencies and discontinuity in the cortex of the bone).
- Tomography, CT scan, MRI scan (rarely).
- Ultrasonography and radioisotope bone scanning. (Bone scan is particularly useful when radiographs/CT scanning are negative in clinically suspect fracture.)

ESSENTIAL MANAGEMENT

General
- Look for shock/haemorrhage and check ABC (see p. 78).
- Look for injury in other areas at risk (head and spine, ribs and pneumothorax, femoral and pelvic injury).

The fracture

Immediate
- Relieve pain (opiates i.v., nerve blocks, splints, traction).
- Establish good i.v. access and send blood for group and crossmatch.
- Open (compound) fractures require debridement, antibiotics and tetanus prophylaxis.

Definitive
- Reduction (closed or open).
- Immobilization (casting, functional bracing, internal fixation, external fixation, traction).
- Rehabilitation (aim to restore the patient to pre-injury level of function with physiotherapy and occupational therapy).

Complications

Early

- Blood loss.
- Infection.
- Fat embolism.
- DVT and PE.
- Renal failure.
- Compartment syndrome.

Late

- Non-union.
- Delayed union.
- Malunion.
- Growth arrest.
- Arthritis.
- Post-traumatic sympathetic (reflex) dystrophy.

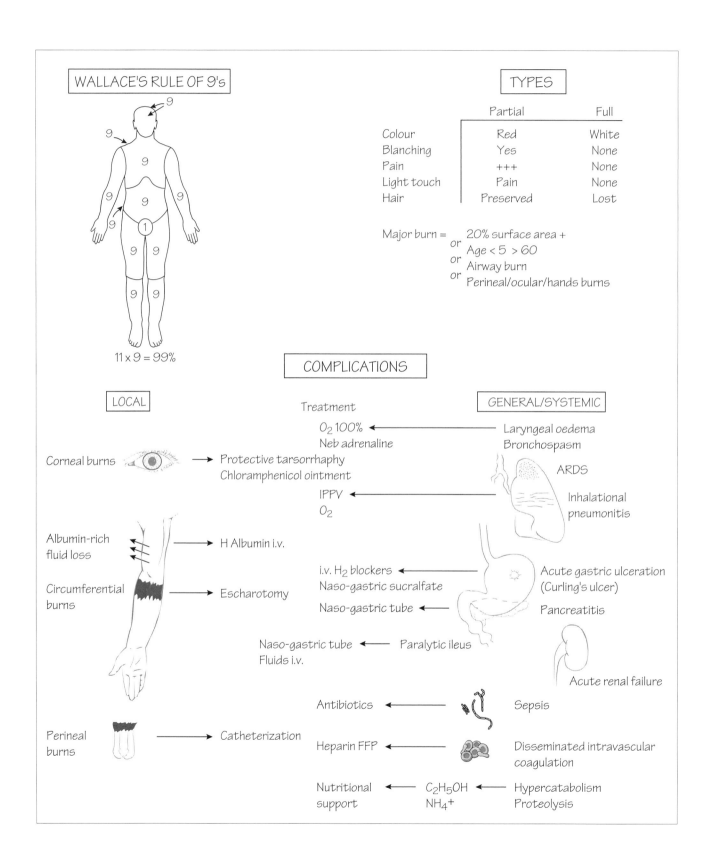

WALLACE'S RULE OF 9's

9

9

9

9 9 9

9 9

1

9 9

9 9

11 x 9 = 99%

TYPES

	Partial	Full
Colour	Red	White
Blanching	Yes	None
Pain	+++	None
Light touch	Pain	None
Hair	Preserved	Lost

Major burn = or { 20% surface area +
Age < 5 > 60
Airway burn
Perineal/ocular/hands burns

COMPLICATIONS

LOCAL

Treatment

GENERAL/SYSTEMIC

O_2 100% ← Laryngeal oedema
Neb adrenaline   Bronchospasm

ARDS

Corneal burns → Protective tarsorrhaphy
Chloramphenicol ointment

IPPV ← Inhalational
O_2 pneumonitis

Albumin-rich → H Albumin i.v.
fluid loss

i.v. H_2 blockers ← Acute gastric ulceration
Naso-gastric sucralfate   (Curling's ulcer)

Circumferential → Escharotomy
burns

Naso-gastric tube ← Pancreatitis

Naso-gastric tube ← Paralytic ileus
Fluids i.v.

Acute renal failure

Antibiotics ← Sepsis

Perineal → Catheterization
burns

Heparin FFP ← Disseminated intravascular
coagulation

Nutritional ← C_2H_5OH ← Hypercatabolism
support NH_4^+ Proteolysis

Definitions

A *burn* is the response of the skin and subcutaneous tissues to thermal injury. A *partial thickness* burn is a burn which either does not destroy the skin epithelium or destroys only part of it. They usually heal with conservative management. A *full thickness* burn destroys all sources of skin epithelial regrowth and may require excision and skin grafting if large.

KEY POINTS
- Start resuscitation immediately in major burns.
- Calculate fluid requirement from the time of the burn.
- Be sure to assess for vital area burns (airway/hands/face/perineum/circumferential).
- Consider referral to a specialist burns centre for all major burns.

Common causes

- Thermal injury from dry (flame, hot metal) or moist (hot liquids or gases) heat sources.
- Electricity (deep burns at entry and exit sites, may cause cardiac arrest).
- Chemicals (usually industrial accidents with acid or alkali).
- Radiation (partial thickness initially, but may progress to chronic deeper injury).

Clinical features

General
- Pain.
- Swelling and blistering.

Specific
- Evidence of smoke inhalation (soot in nose or sputum, burns in the mouth, hoarseness).
- Eye or eyelid burns (early ophthalmological opinion).
- Circumferential burns (will need escharotomy).

Investigations

- FBC.
- U+E.
- If inhalation suspected: chest X-ray, arterial blood gases, CO estimation.
- Blood group and crossmatch.
- ECG/cardiac enzymes with electrical burns.

Complications

Immediate
Compartment syndrome from circumferential burns (limb burns → limb ischaemia, thoracic burns → hypoxia from restrictive respiratory failure) (prevent by urgent escharotomy).

Early
- Hyperkalaemia (from cytolysis in large burns). Treat with insulin and dextrose.
- Acute renal failure (combination of hypovolaemia, sepsis, tissue toxins). Prevent by aggressive early resuscitation, ensuring high GFR with fluid loading and diuretics, treat sepsis.
- Infection (beware of *Streptococcus*). Treat established infection (10^6 organisms present in wound biopsy) with systemic antibiotics.
- Stress ulceration (Curling's ulcer) (prevent with antacid, H_2-blocker or proton pump inhibitor prophylaxis).

Late
Contractures.

ESSENTIAL MANAGEMENT

General
- Start resuscitation (ABC (see p. 78), set up good i.v. lines, give O_2).
- Assess size of burn (Wallace's rule of 9s).

Major burns (>20% burn in adult, >10% in child)
- Monitor pulse, BP, temperature, urinary output, give adequate analgesia i.v., consider nasogastric tube, give tetanus prophylaxis.
- Give i.v. fluids according to Muir–Barclay formula:
  % burn × wt in kg/2 = one aliquot of fluid.
  Give six aliquots of fluid over first 36 h in 4, 4, 4, 6, 6, 12-hour sequence from time of burn. Colloid, albumin or plasma solutions are used.
- The burn wound is treated as for minor burns (see below).
- Consider referral to a burns centre.

Minor burns (<20% burn in adult, <10% in child)
- Treatment by exposure—debride wound and leave exposed in special clean environment.
- Treatment by dressings—cover with tulle gras impregnated with chlorhexidine or silver sulphadiazine under absorptive gauze dressings.
- Debridement of eschar and split skin grafting.

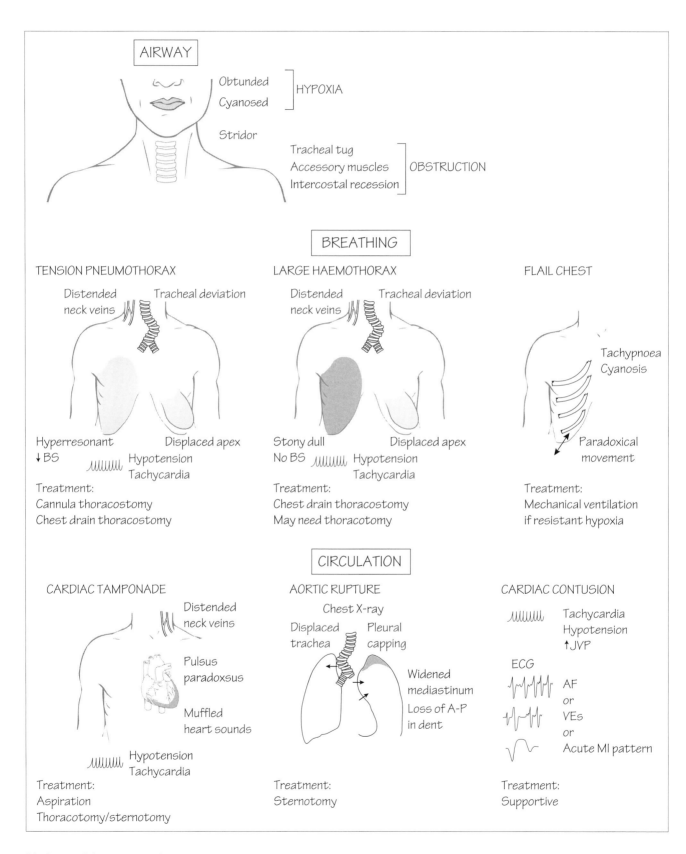

AIRWAY

Obtunded
Cyanosed   ] HYPOXIA

Stridor

Tracheal tug
Accessory muscles   ] OBSTRUCTION
Intercostal recession

BREATHING

TENSION PNEUMOTHORAX

Distended   Tracheal deviation
neck veins

Hyperresonant   Displaced apex
↓ BS   Hypotension
               Tachycardia
Treatment:
Cannula thoracostomy
Chest drain thoracostomy

LARGE HAEMOTHORAX

Distended   Tracheal deviation
neck veins

Stony dull   Displaced apex
No BS   Hypotension
               Tachycardia
Treatment:
Chest drain thoracostomy
May need thoracotomy

FLAIL CHEST

Tachypnoea
Cyanosis

Paradoxical
movement

Treatment:
Mechanical ventilation
if resistant hypoxia

CIRCULATION

CARDIAC TAMPONADE

Distended
neck veins

Pulsus
paradoxsus

Muffled
heart sounds

Hypotension
Tachycardia
Treatment:
Aspiration
Thoracotomy/sternotomy

AORTIC RUPTURE

Chest X-ray
Displaced   Pleural
trachea   capping

Widened
mediastinum
Loss of A-P
in dent

Treatment:
Sternotomy

CARDIAC CONTUSION

Tachycardia
Hypotension
↑JVP

ECG

AF
or
VEs
or
Acute MI pattern

Treatment:
Supportive

Definition

Major trauma (MT) can be defined as injury (or injuries) of organs of severity sufficient to present an immediate threat to life. MT often involves multiple injuries. The majority of patients who reach hospital alive following MT have potentially survivable injuries if detected and treated early.

KEY POINTS
- Treat all MT patients as having a potentially unstable cervical spine.
- Treat life-threatening injuries identified in the primary survey immediately upon discovery.
- Undiagnosed hypotension is due to occult haemorrhage unless proven otherwise.
- Emergency surgery may be part of the resuscitation of patients suffering from internal haemorrhage.

Principles of management

Management for MT is divided into two categories.
- **'First aid'**—'roadside' given by paramedics or on-site medical teams. Aims to maintain life during extraction and evacuation of patient.
- **Primary survey**—in hospital performed by A&E or Trauma Teams. Aims to identify and treat life-threatening injuries to airways, respiratory and cardiovascular systems and perform major skeletal radiology. Known as the ABC(DE) **secondary survey**—in hospital performed by A&E or Trauma Teams, possibly with specialist surgical staff. Aims to identify and assess all major injuries.

Patterns of injury

Some of the major injuries which may be encountered in the primary survey are shown opposite. Mechanisms of injury and patterns of injury may be associated, e.g.

Restrained RTA	Pedestrian collision
Cervical spine injury	Long bone fractures
Sternal fracture	Knee ligamentous injury
Cardiac contusion	Rib fractures
Liver laceration	Pneumothorax
	Facial fractures
	Head injury

ESSENTIAL PRIMARY SURVEY MANAGEMENT

Cervical spine
- Stabilize with in-line manual traction.
- Secure with hard collar, head supports and tape.
- Can only be 'cleared' by normal examination in a fully conscious patient or normal X-rays.

Lateral C spine/X-ray (must include C7–T1)

A Airway management (see opposite for major abnormalities)
- Clear obstructions by hand and lift chin (obtunded patients).
- Secure airway with oropharyngeal or nasopharyngeal airway (obtunded patients).
- Definitive airway (direct access to intratracheal oxygenation) indicated by:
  Apnoea / (risk of) upper airway obstruction / (risk of) aspiration / need for mechanical ventilation.
  Orotracheal tube.
  Nasotracheal tube.
- Surgical airway (cricothyroidotomy) indicated by:
  Maxillofacial injuries / laryngeal disruption / failure to intubate.

B Breathing (see opposite for some major abnormalities)
- Administer supplemental O_2.
- Assess respiratory rate / air entry (symmetry) / chest wall motion (symmetry) / tracheal position.
- Monitor with pulse oximetry and observations.

CXR

C Circulation (see opposite for some major abnormalities)
- Assess pulse rate and character / blood pressure / apex beat / JVP / heart sounds / evidence of blood loss.
- Draw blood for Cross-match, FBC and U+E.

Pelvic X-ray

D Dysfunction of the CNS
- Assess GCS (see p. 81) / pupil reactivity / limb gross motor and sensory function where possible.

E Exposure of extremities
- Assess limbs for major long bone injuries and sites of major blood loss.

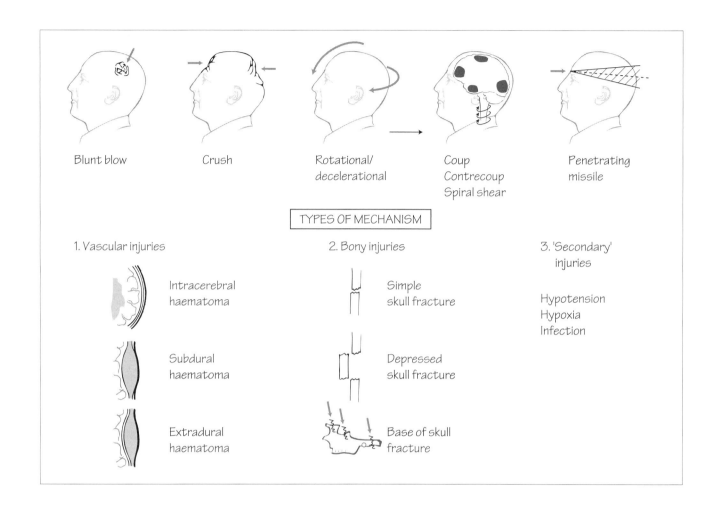

Blunt blow   Crush   Rotational/decelerational   Coup Contrecoup Spiral shear   Penetrating missile

TYPES OF MECHANISM

1. Vascular injuries

Intracerebral haematoma

Subdural haematoma

Extradural haematoma

2. Bony injuries

Simple skull fracture

Depressed skull fracture

Base of skull fracture

3. 'Secondary' injuries

Hypotension
Hypoxia
Infection

Definitions

• A *head injury* is the process whereby direct or decelerating trauma to the head results in skull and brain damage.
• *Primary brain injury* is the damage that occurs to the brain immediately as the result of the trauma.
• *Secondary brain injury* is the damage that develops later as a result of complications.

Epidemiology

Head injury is very common. A million patients each year present to A&E departments in the UK with head injury and about 5000 patients die each year following head injuries.

Pathophysiology

Direct blow

May cause damage to the brain at the site of the blow (*coup injury*) or to the side opposite the blow when the brain moves within the skull and hits the opposite wall (*contrecoup injury*).

Rotation/deceleration

Neck flexion, extension or rotation results in the brain striking bony points within the skull (e.g. the wing of the sphenoid bone). Severe rotation also causes shear injuries within the white matter of the brain and brainstem, causing axonal injury and intracerebral petechial haemorrhages.

Crush

The brain is often remarkably spared direct injury unless severe (especially in children with elastic skulls).

Missiles

Tend to cause loss of tissue with injury proportionate. Brain swelling less of a problem due to the skull disruption automatically decompressing the brain!
• The degree of primary brain injury is directly related to the amount of force applied to the head.
• Secondary damage results from: respiratory complications (*hypoxia, hypercarbia, airway obstruction*), hypovolaemic shock (head injury does not cause hypovolaemic shock—look for another cause), intracranial bleeding, cerebral oedema, epilepsy, infection and hydrocephalus.

Clinical features

• History of direct trauma to head or deceleration.
• Patient must be assessed fully for other injuries.
• Level of consciousness determined by GCS.

The Glasgow Coma Scale.

Eye opening	Voice response	Best motor response
Spontaneous 4	Alert and orientated 5	Obeys commands 6
To voice 3	Confused 4	Localizes pain 5
To pain 2	Inappropriate 3	Flexes to pain 4
No eye opening 1	Incomprehensible 2	Abnormal flexion to pain 3
	No voice response 1	Extends to pain 2
		No response to pain 1

Fully conscious: GCS = 15; deep coma: GCS = 3.

• Pupillary inequalities or abnormal light reflex indicate intracranial haemorrhage.
• Headache, nausea, vomiting, a falling pulse rate and rising BP indicate cerebral oedema.

Investigations

• Skull X-ray: AP, lateral and Towne's views.
• CT/MRI scan: show contusions, haematomas, hydrocephalus, cerebral oedema.

Head injury/2

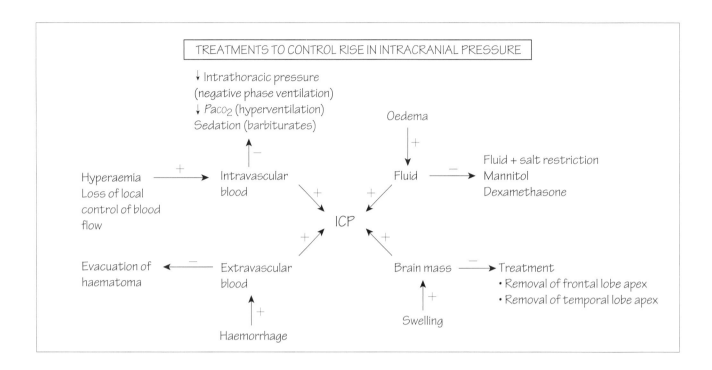

Complications
Skull fractures

Indicate severity of injury. No specific treatment required unless compound, depressed or associated with chronic CSF loss (e.g. anterior cranial fossa basal skull fracture).

Intracranial haemorrhage

- Extradural haemorrhage: tear in middle meningeal artery. Haematoma between skull and dura. Often a 'lucid interval' before signs of raised intracranial pressure (ICP) ensue (falling pulse, rising BP, ipsilateral pupillary dilatation, contralateral paresis or paralysis). Treatment is by evacuation of haematoma via burr holes.
- Acute subdural haemorrhage: tearing of veins between arachnoid and dura mater. Usually seen in elderly. Progressive neurological deterioration. Treatment is by evacuation but even then recovery may be incomplete.
- Chronic subdural haematoma: tear in vein leads to subdural haematoma which enlarges slowly by absorption of CSF. Often the precipitating injury is trivial. Drowsiness and confusion, headache, hemiplegia. Treatment is by evacuation of the clot.
- Intracerebral haemorrhage: haemorrhage into brain substance causes irreversible damage. Efforts are made to avoid secondary injury by ensuring adequate oxygenation and nutrition.

Prognosis

Prognosis is related to level of consciousness on arrival in hospital.

GCS on admission	Mortality
15	1%
8–12	5%
<8	40%

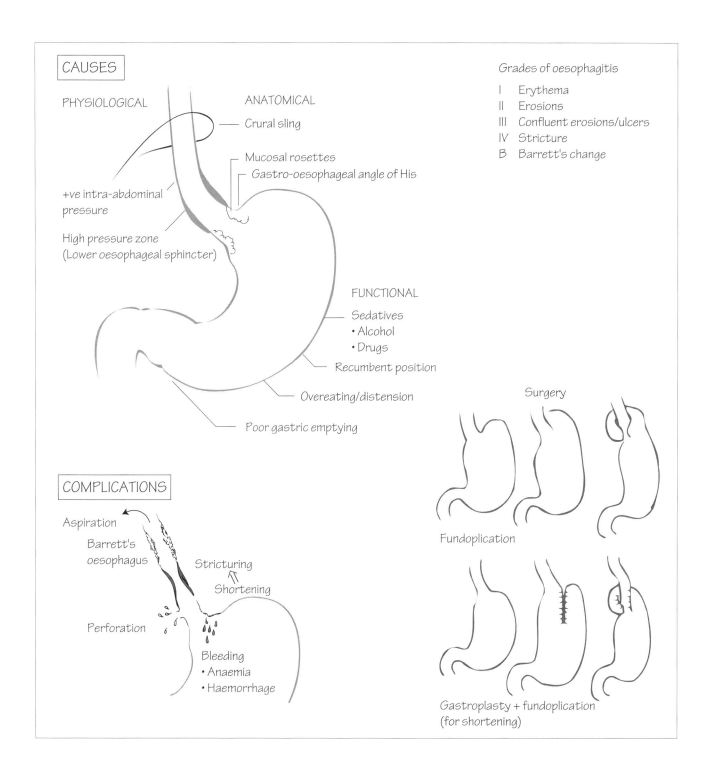

CAUSES

PHYSIOLOGICAL

ANATOMICAL

Crural sling

Mucosal rosettes
Gastro-oesophageal angle of His

+ve intra-abdominal pressure

High pressure zone
(Lower oesophageal sphincter)

FUNCTIONAL

Sedatives
• Alcohol
• Drugs

Recumbent position

Overeating/distension

Poor gastric emptying

Grades of oesophagitis

I   Erythema
II   Erosions
III Confluent erosions/ulcers
IV   Stricture
B   Barrett's change

COMPLICATIONS

Aspiration

Barrett's oesophagus

Stricturing
Shortening

Perforation

Bleeding
• Anaemia
• Haemorrhage

Surgery

Fundoplication

Gastroplasty + fundoplication
(for shortening)

Definitions

Gastro-oesophageal reflux is a condition caused by the retrograde passage of gastric contents into the oesophagus resulting in inflammation (*oesophagitis*), which manifests as dyspepsia. A *hiatus hernia* is an abnormal protrusion of the proximal stomach through the oesophageal opening in the diaphragm resulting in a more proximal positioning of the oesophagogastric junction and predisposition to gastro-oesophageal reflux disease (GORD). *Sliding* (common) and *rolling* or *para-oesophageal* (rare) hiatus hernias are recognized.

KEY POINTS

• The majority of GORD is benign and uncomplicated.
• Barrett's oesophagus is an increasingly recognized association predisposing to adenocarcinoma of the oesophagus.
• Patients over the 45 years or with suspicious symptoms should have malignancy excluded as a cause when first presenting with GORD symptoms.
• Surgery for GORD should be reserved for complications or patients resistant to medical therapy.

Common causes

• Failure of normal mechanisms of gastro-oesophageal continence (LOS pressure, length of intra-abdominal LOS, angle of His, sling fibres around the cardia, the crural fibres of the diaphragm, the mucosal rosette).
• LOS pressure reduced by smoking, alcohol and coffee.

Clinical features

• Retrosternal burning pain, radiating to epigastrium, jaw and arms. (Oesophageal pain is often confused with cardiac pain.)
• Regurgitation of acid contents into the mouth (waterbrash).
• Back pain (a penetrating ulcer in Barrett's oesophagus).
• Dysphagia from a benign stricture.

Investigations

• Barium swallow and meal: sliding hiatus hernia, oesophageal ulcer, stricture.
• Oesophagoscopy: assess oesophagitis, biopsy for histology, dilate stricture if present.
• 24-hour pH monitoring: assess the degree of reflux.
• Oesophageal manometry.

ESSENTIAL MANAGEMENT

General
• Lose weight, avoid smoking, coffee, alcohol and chocolate.
• Avoid tight garments and stooping.

Medical
• Exclude carcinoma by OGD in patients over 45 years and with symptoms suspicious of malignancy.
• Control acid secretion (H_2 receptor antagonists (e.g. ranitidine) or proton pump inhibitors (PPIs) (e.g. omeprazole)).
• Minimize effects of reflux (give alginates to protect oesophagus).
• Prokinetic agents (e.g. metoclopramide, cisapride) improve LOS tone and promote gastric emptying.

Surgical
• Anti-reflux surgery (e.g. Nissen fundoplication) which may be performed by laparotomy or laparoscopy. Indicated for:
   complications of reflux;
   failed medical control of symptoms;
   ?long-term dependence on medical treatment;
   ?'large volume' reflux.

Complications

• Benign stricture of the oesophagus.
• Barrett's oesophagus (see below).
• Bleeding.

Barrett's oesophagus

Definition and aetiology

>3 cm of columnar epithelium lining the lower anatomical oesophagus. May be related to eradication of *H. pylori* and increasing incidence of GORD.

Diagnosis

Can only be confidently made by biopsy but appearances of 'reddish' mucosa in the lower oesophagus are typical on OGD.

Complications

Risk of adenocarcinoma:
• 2%—no dysplasia present;
• 20%—low-grade dysplasia present;
• 50%—high-grade dysplasia present.

Treatment

• Follow-up OGD (close surveillance if low-grade dysplasia) and PPI/H_2 blockers.
• Oesophagectomy if high-grade dysplasia due to risk of carcinoma.

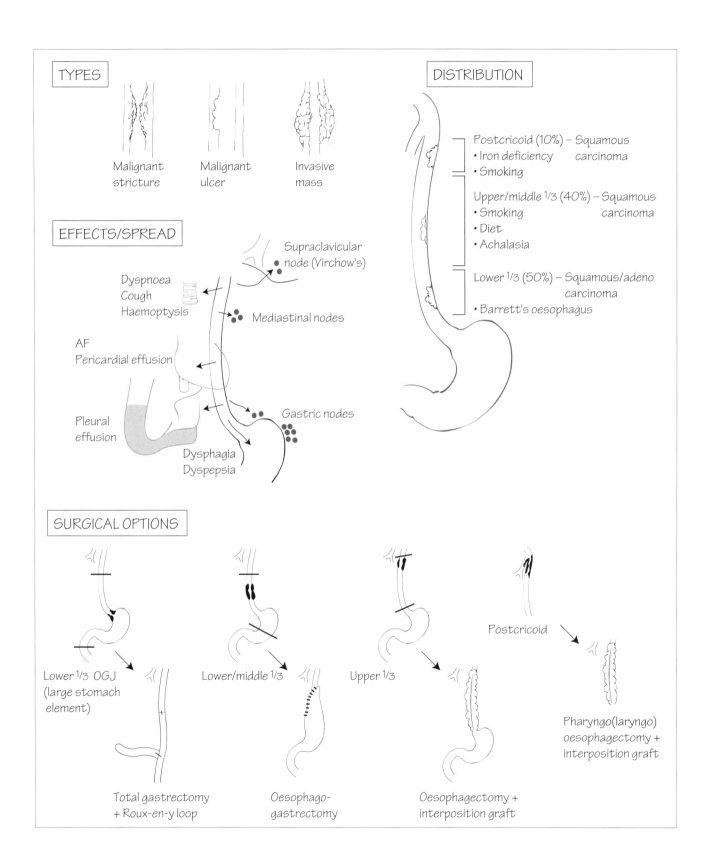

TYPES

Malignant stricture

Malignant ulcer

Invasive mass

EFFECTS/SPREAD

Supraclavicular node (Virchow's)

Dyspnoea
Cough
Haemoptysis

Mediastinal nodes

AF
Pericardial effusion

Pleural effusion

Gastric nodes

Dysphagia
Dyspepsia

DISTRIBUTION

Postcricoid (10%) – Squamous carcinoma
• Iron deficiency
• Smoking

Upper/middle 1/3 (40%) – Squamous carcinoma
• Smoking
• Diet
• Achalasia

Lower 1/3 (50%) – Squamous/adeno carcinoma
• Barrett's oesophagus

SURGICAL OPTIONS

Lower 1/3 OGJ (large stomach element)

Total gastrectomy + Roux-en-y loop

Lower/middle 1/3

Oesophago-gastrectomy

Upper 1/3

Oesophagectomy + interposition graft

Postcricoid

Pharyngo(laryngo) oesophagectomy + interposition graft

Definition

Malignant lesion of the epithelial lining of the oesophagus.

> **KEY POINTS**
> - All new symptoms of dysphagia should raise the possibility of oesophageal carcinoma.
> - Adenocarcinoma of the oesophagus is increasingly common.
> - Only a minority of tumours are successfully cured by surgery.

Epidemiology

- Male/female 3 : 1, peak incidence 50–70 years. High incidence in areas of China, Russia, Scandinavia and among the Bantu in South Africa.
- Adenocarcinoma has the fastest increasing incidence of any carcinoma in the UK.

Aetiology

The following are predisposing factors.
- Alcohol consumption and cigarette smoking.
- Chronic oesophagitis and Barrett's oesophagus.
- Stricture from corrosive (lye) oesophagitis.
- Achalasia.
- Plummer–Vinson syndrome (oesophageal web, mucosal lesions of mouth and pharynx, iron deficiency anaemia).
- Nitrosamines.

Pathology

- Histological type: 90% squamous carcinoma (upper two-thirds of oesophagus); 10% adenocarcinoma (lower third of oesophagus).
- Spread: lymphatics, direct extension, vascular invasion.

Clinical features

- Dysphagia progressing from solids to liquids.
- Weight loss and weakness.
- Aspiration pneumonia.

Investigations

- Barium swallow: narrowed lumen with 'shouldering'.
- Oesophagoscopy and biopsy: malignant stricture. (Transluminal ultrasound may help assess local invasion.)
- Bronchoscopy: assess bronchial invasion with upper third lesions.
- CT scanning (helical): assess degree of spread if surgery is being contemplated.
- Laparoscopy to assess liver and peritoneal involvement prior to proceeding to surgery.

ESSENTIAL MANAGEMENT

Palliation
- Intubation with Atkinson or Celestine tube or expanding endoprosthesis.
- Intraluminal irradiation with iridium wires.
- Laser resection of the tumour to create lumen.
- Surgical excision of the tumour.

Curative treatment
Surgical resection is curative only if lymph nodes are not involved. Reconstruction is by gastric 'pull-up' or colon interposition.

Other treatment
Combination therapy with external beam radiation, chemotherapy and surgery is under trial and probably indicated for squamous carcinoma.

Prognosis

Following resection, 5-year survival rates are about 15%, but overall 5-year survival (palliation and resection) is only about 4%.

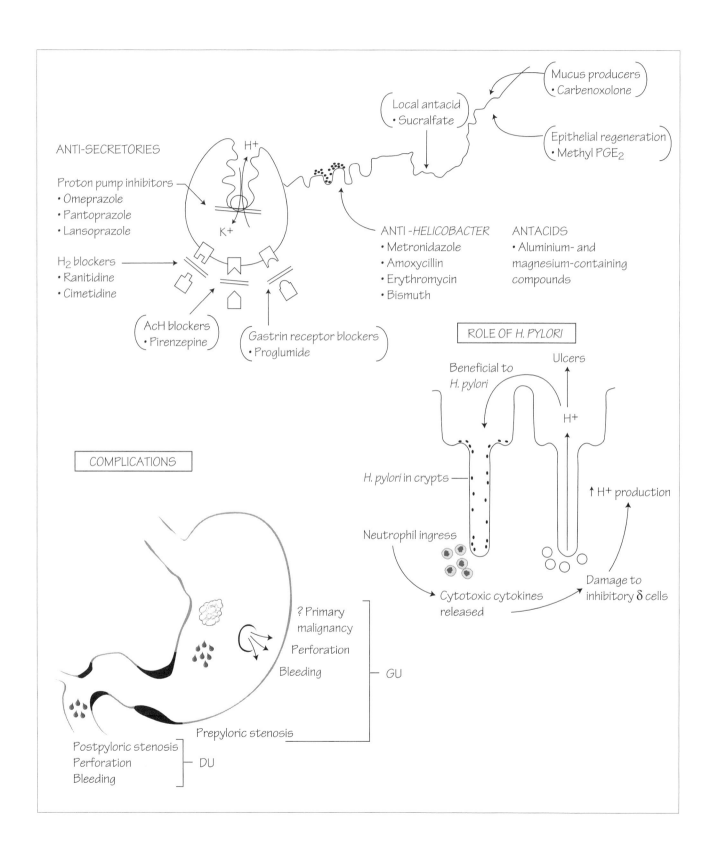

ANTI-SECRETORIES

Proton pump inhibitors
• Omeprazole
• Pantoprazole
• Lansoprazole

H_2 blockers
• Ranitidine
• Cimetidine

AcH blockers
• Pirenzepine

Gastrin receptor blockers
• Proglumide

H^+

K^+

Local antacid
• Sucralfate

Mucus producers
• Carbenoxolone

Epithelial regeneration
• Methyl PGE_2

ANTI -HELICOBACTER
• Metronidazole
• Amoxycillin
• Erythromycin
• Bismuth

ANTACIDS
• Aluminium- and magnesium-containing compounds

ROLE OF H. PYLORI

Beneficial to H. pylori

Ulcers

H^+

H. pylori in crypts

↑ H^+ production

Neutrophil ingress

Cytotoxic cytokines released

Damage to inhibitory δ cells

COMPLICATIONS

? Primary malignancy

Perforation

Bleeding

GU

Prepyloric stenosis

Postpyloric stenosis
Perforation
Bleeding

DU

Definition

A peptic ulcer is a break in the epithelial surface of the oesophagus, stomach or duodenum (rarely Meckel's diverticulum) caused by the action of gastric secretions (acid and pepsin) and, in the case of duodenal ulceration, infection with *H. pylori*.

> **KEY POINTS**
> - Not all dyspepsia is due to PUD.
> - The majority of chronic duodenal ulcers are related to *H. Pylori* infection and respond to eradication therapy.
> - All patients over 45 at presentation or with suspicious symptoms require endoscopy to exclude malignancy.
> - Surgery is usually limited to complications of ulcer disease and failure of compliant medical therapy.

Common causes

- Imbalance between acid/pepsin secretion and mucosal defence.
- Acid hypersecretion occurs because of increased numbers of parietal cells (or rarely in response to gastrin hypersecretion in the Zollinger–Ellison syndrome).
- Defects in mucosal defence (e.g. mucus secretion).
- NSAIDs and the usual suspects: alcohol, cigarettes and 'stress'!
- Infection with *H. pylori*.

Clinical features

Duodenal ulcer and type II gastric ulcer (i.e. prepyloric and antral)

- Male/female 4 : 1, peak incidence 25–50 years.
- Epigastric pain during fasting (hunger pain), relieved by food/antacids, typically exhibits periodicity.
- Boring back pain if ulcer is penetrating posteriorly.
- Haematemesis from ulcer penetrating gastroduodenal artery posteriorly.
- Peritonitis if perforation occurs with anterior duodenal ulcer.
- Vomiting if gastric outlet obstruction (pyloric stenosis) occurs (note succussion splash and watch for hypokalaemic, hypochloraemic alkalosis).

Type I gastric ulcer (i.e. body of stomach)

- Male/female 3 : 1, peak incidence 50+ years.
- Epigastric pain induced by eating.

- Weight loss.
- Nausea and vomiting.
- Anaemia from chronic blood loss.

Investigations

- FBC: to check for anaemia.
- U+E: rarely indicates Zollinger–Ellison syndrome.
- Faecal occult blood.
- OGD: necessary to exclude malignant gastric ulcer in:
  patients over 45 at first presentation;
  concomitant anaemia;
  short history of symptoms;
  other symptoms suggestive of malignancy.
- Useful to obtain biopsy for *Campylobacter*-like organism (CLO) (urease) test.
- Barium meal: best for patients unable to tolerate OGD or evaluation of the duodenum in cases of pyloric stenosis.
- Urease breath test/*H. pylori* serology: non-invasive method of assessing the presence of *H. pylori* infection. Used to direct therapy or confirm eradication.

ESSENTIAL MANAGEMENT

Medical
- Avoid smoking and foods that cause pain.
- Antacids for symptomatic relief.
- H₂ blockers (ranitidine, cimetidine).
- PPIs (omeprazole).
- Colloidal bismuth.
- Ampicillin or tetracycline + metronidazole.
(These are effective against *Helicobacter pylori*.)
- Re-endoscope patients with gastric ulcer after 6 weeks because of risk of malignancy.

Surgical
- Only indicated for failure of medical treatment and complications.
- Elective for duodenal ulcer: highly selective vagotomy; rarely performed now.
- Elective for gastric ulcer: Billroth I gastrectomy.
- Perforated duodenal/gastric ulcer: simple closure of perforation and biopsy.
- Haemorrhage: endoscopic control by sclerotherapy, undersewing bleeding vessel ± vagotomy.
- Pyloric stenosis: gastroenterostomy ± truncal vagotomy.

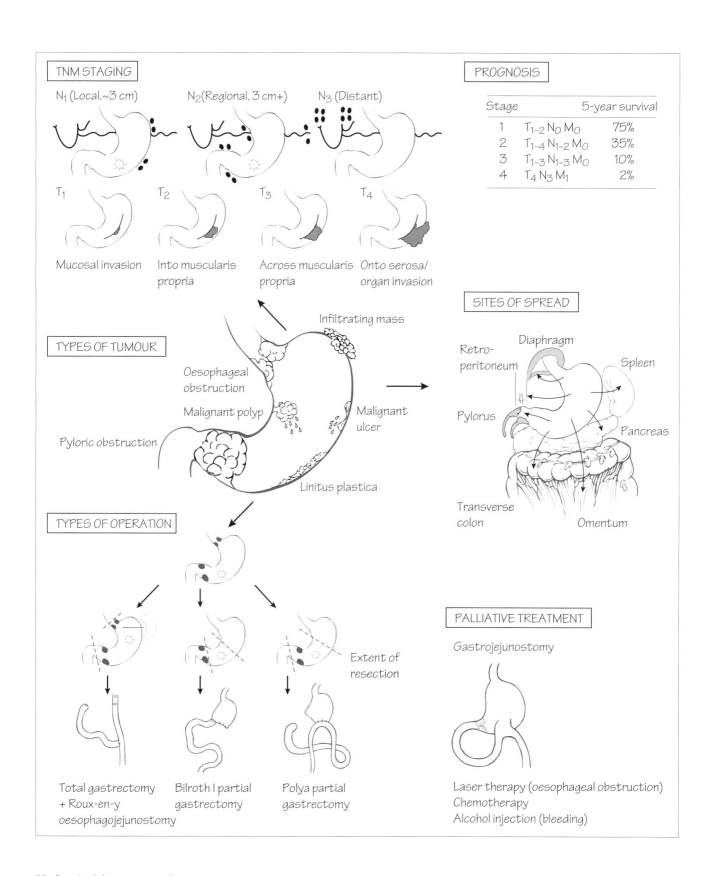

TNM STAGING

N_1 (Local, ~3 cm) N_2 (Regional, 3 cm+) N_3 (Distant)

T_1 T_2 T_3 T_4

Mucosal invasion | Into muscularis propria | Across muscularis propria | Onto serosa/organ invasion

PROGNOSIS

Stage		5-year survival
1	$T_{1-2} N_0 M_0$	75%
2	$T_{1-4} N_{1-2} M_0$	35%
3	$T_{1-3} N_{1-3} M_0$	10%
4	$T_4 N_3 M_1$	2%

TYPES OF TUMOUR

Infiltrating mass

Oesophageal obstruction

Malignant polyp

Pyloric obstruction

Malignant ulcer

Linitus plastica

SITES OF SPREAD

Retro-peritoneum   Diaphragm   Spleen

Pylorus   Pancreas

Transverse colon   Omentum

TYPES OF OPERATION

Extent of resection

Total gastrectomy + Roux-en-y oesophagojejunostomy | Bilroth I partial gastrectomy | Polya partial gastrectomy

PALLIATIVE TREATMENT

Gastrojejunostomy

Laser therapy (oesophageal obstruction)
Chemotherapy
Alcohol injection (bleeding)

Definition

Malignant lesion of the stomach epithelium.

> **KEY POINTS**
> • The majority of tumours are unresectable at presentation.
> • Tumours considered candidates for resection should be staged with CT and laparoscopy to reduce the risk of an 'open and shut' laparotomy.
> • Most tumours are poorly responsive to chemotherapy.

Epidemiology

Male/female 2 : 1, peak incidence 50+ years. Incidence has decreased in Western world over last 50 years. Still common in Japan, Chile and Scandinavia.

Aetiology

The following are predisposing factors.
• Diet (smoked fish, pickled vegetables, benzpyrene, nitrosamines).
• Atrophic gastritis.
• Pernicious anaemia.
• Previous partial gastrectomy.
• Familial hypogammaglobulinaemia.
• Gastric adenomatous polyps.
• Blood group A.

Pathology

• Histology: adenocarcinoma.
• Advanced gastric cancer (penetrated muscularis propria) may be polypoid, ulcerating or infiltrating (i.e. linitus plastica).
• Early gastric cancer (confined to mucosa or submucosa).
• Spread: lymphatic (e.g. Virchow's node); haematogenous to liver, lung, brain; transcoelomic to ovary (Krukenberg tumour).

Clinical features

• History of recent dyspepsia (epigastric discomfort, postprandial fullness, loss of appetite).
• Anaemia.
• Dysphagia.
• Vomiting.
• Weight loss.
• The presence of physical signs usually indicates advanced (incurable) disease.

Investigations

• FBC.
• U+E.
• LFTs.
• OGD (see the lesion and obtain biopsy to distinguish from benign gastric ulcer).
• Barium meal (space-occupying lesion/ulcer with rolled edge). Best for patients unable to tolerate OGD.
• CT scan (helical): stages disease locally and systemically.
• Laparoscopy: used to exclude undiagnosed peritoneal or liver secondaries prior to consideration of resection.

> **ESSENTIAL MANAGEMENT**
> • Palliation (metastatic disease or gross distal nodal disease at presentation):
>   gastrectomy: local symptoms, e.g. bleeding;
>   gastroenterostomy: malignant pyloric obstruction;
>   intubation: obstructing lesions at the cardia.
> • Curative treatment (resectable primary and local nodes).
> • Surgical excision with clear margins and locoregional lymph node clearance (D2 gastrectomy).
> • Other treatment: combination chemotherapy with etoposide, adriamycin and cisplatin may induce regression.

Prognosis

Following 'curative' resection, 5-year survival rates are approximately 20%, but overall 5-year survival (palliation and resection) is only about 5%.

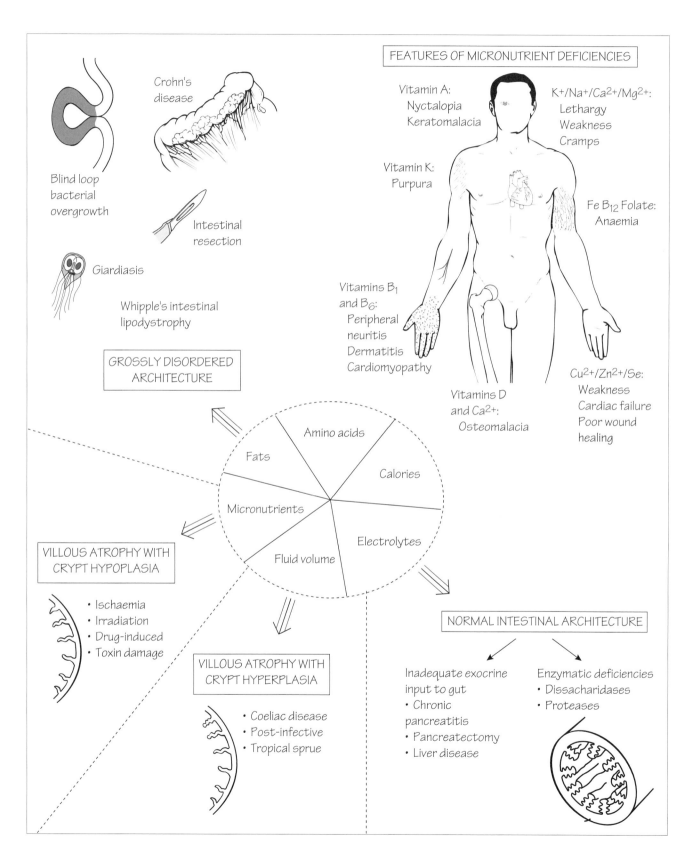

Crohn's disease

Blind loop bacterial overgrowth

Intestinal resection

Giardiasis

Whipple's intestinal lipodystrophy

GROSSLY DISORDERED ARCHITECTURE

FEATURES OF MICRONUTRIENT DEFICIENCIES

Vitamin A:
Nyctalopia
Keratomalacia

$K^+/Na^+/Ca^{2+}/Mg^{2+}$:
Lethargy
Weakness
Cramps

Vitamin K:
Purpura

Fe B_{12} Folate:
Anaemia

Vitamins B_1 and B_6:
Peripheral neuritis
Dermatitis
Cardiomyopathy

Vitamins D and Ca^{2+}:
Osteomalacia

$Cu^{2+}/Zn^{2+}/Se$:
Weakness
Cardiac failure
Poor wound healing

Amino acids

Fats

Calories

Micronutrients

Electrolytes

Fluid volume

VILLOUS ATROPHY WITH CRYPT HYPOPLASIA

• Ischaemia
• Irradiation
• Drug-induced
• Toxin damage

VILLOUS ATROPHY WITH CRYPT HYPERPLASIA

• Coeliac disease
• Post-infective
• Tropical sprue

NORMAL INTESTINAL ARCHITECTURE

Inadequate exocrine input to gut
• Chronic pancreatitis
• Pancreatectomy
• Liver disease

Enzymatic deficiencies
• Dissacharidases
• Proteases

Definition

Malabsorption is the failure of the body to acquire and conserve adequate amounts of one or more essential dietary elements. The cause may be localized or generalized.

> **KEY POINTS**
> - Malabsorption usually affects several nutrient groups.
> - Coeliac disease is a common cause and may present with obscure, vague abdominal symptoms.
> - Always consider micronutrients and trace elements in malabsorption.

Differential diagnosis

Coeliac disease

- Classically presents as sensitivity to gluten-containing foods with diarrhoea, steatorrhoea and weight loss in early adulthood.
- Mild forms may present later in life with non-specific symptoms of malaise, anaemia (including iron deficiency picture), abdominal cramps and weight loss.

Crohn's disease

- Commonest presenting symptoms are colicky abdominal pains with diarrhoea and weight loss.
- Malabsorption is an uncommon presenting symptom but often accompanies stenosing or inflammatory complications of widespread ileal disease.

Intestinal resection

- Global malabsorption may develop after small bowel resections leaving less than 50 cm of functional ileum. Water and electrolyte balance is most disordered but fat, vitamin and other nutrient absorption is also affected with lengths progressively less than 50 cm.
- Specific malabsorption may result from relatively small resection (e.g. fat and vitamin B12 malabsorption after terminal ileal resection, vitamin B12 and iron malabsorption after gastrectomy).

Whipple's disease (intestinal lipodystrophy)

- Fat malabsorption caused by intestinal infection blocking the lacteals with macrophages and bacteria.
- Presents with steatorrhoea associated with arthralgia and malaise.

Bacterial overgrowth

- Malabsorption caused by bacterial metabolism of nutrients and production of breakdown products such as CO_2 and H_2.
- Usually a result of exclusion of a loop of ileum (e.g. in Crohn's disease, postsurgery, intestinal fistulation) with consequent bacterial overgrowth, although can occur in chronically damaged or dilated bowel.

Radiation enteropathy

- Slow onset, progressive global malabsorption. Usually only if large areas of ileum affected.
- May occur many years after original radiotherapy exposure.

Chronic ischaemic enteropathy

Rare cause of malabsorption. Usually accompanied by chronic intestinal ischaemia causing 'mesenteric angina/claudication' upon eating.

Parasitic infection

Common in tropics but rare in the UK.

Key investigations

- FBC, U+E, LFTs: general nutritional status.
- Trace elements (Zn, Se, Mg, Mn, Cu).
- Anti a-gliadin antibodies (serum assay for coeliac disease).
- Small bowel meal or enema: best for Crohn's disease, radiation or ischaemic enteropathy and blind loop formation.

> **ESSENTIAL MANAGEMENT**
> - Major deficiencies should be corrected by supplementation (oral or parenteral).
> - Infectious causes should be excluded or (consider probiotics) treated promptly.
> - Coeliac disease: gluten-free diet.
> - Crohn's disease: usually requires resection of affected segment. Course of systemic steroids or immunosuppressive agents may help.
> - Radiation or ischaemic malabsorption rarely responds to any medical therapy—often requires parenteral nutrition.

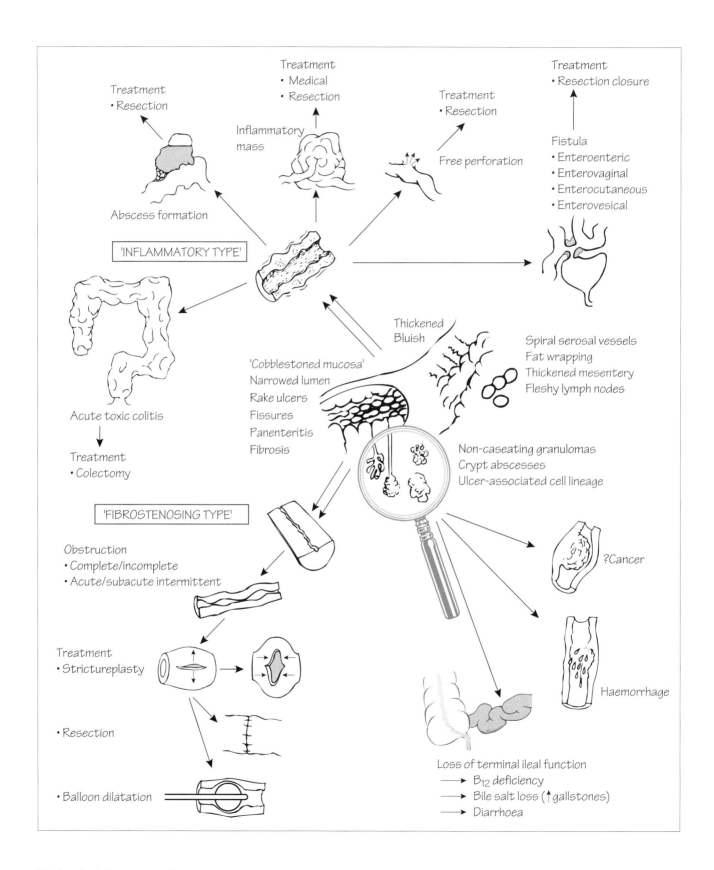

Treatment
• Resection

Treatment
• Medical
• Resection

Inflammatory
mass

Treatment
• Resection

Treatment
• Resection closure

Fistula
• Enteroenteric
• Enterovaginal
• Enterocutaneous
• Enterovesical

Free perforation

Abscess formation

'INFLAMMATORY TYPE'

Thickened
Bluish

Spiral serosal vessels
Fat wrapping
Thickened mesentery
Fleshy lymph nodes

Acute toxic colitis

'Cobblestoned mucosa'
Narrowed lumen
Rake ulcers
Fissures
Panenteritis
Fibrosis

Non-caseating granulomas
Crypt abscesses
Ulcer-associated cell lineage

Treatment
• Colectomy

'FIBROSTENOSING TYPE'

?Cancer

Obstruction
• Complete/incomplete
• Acute/subacute intermittent

Treatment
• Strictureplasty

• Resection

Haemorrhage

• Balloon dilatation

Loss of terminal ileal function
⟶ B_{12} deficiency
⟶ Bile salt loss (↑gallstones)
⟶ Diarrhoea

Definition

Crohn's disease is a chronic transmural inflammatory disorder of the alimentary tract.

Epidemiology

Male/female 1 : 1.6. Young adults. High incidence among Europeans and Jewish people.

Aetiology

- Unknown.
- Impaired cell-mediated immunity.
- Genetic link probable but candidate genes unknown.
- No proven link to mycobacterial infection or measles virus hypersensitivity.
- Smoking associated with recurrence.

Pathology

Macroscopic

- May affect any part of the alimentary tract.
- Skip lesions in bowel (affected bowel wall and mesentery are thickened and oedematous, frequent fistulae).
- Affected bowel characteristically 'fat wrapped' by mesenteric fat.
- Perianal disease characterized by perianal induration and sepsis with fissure, sinus and fistula formation.

Histology

- Transmural inflammation in the form of lymphoid aggregates.
- Non-caseating epithelioid cell granulomas with Langhans giant cells. Regional nodes may also be involved.

Clinical features

Acute presentations (uncommon)

- RIF peritonitis (like appendicitis picture).
- Generalized peritonitis (due to free perforation).

Subacute presentations (common)

- RIF inflammatory mass (usually associated with fistulae or abscess formation).
- Widespread ileal inflammation—general ill health, malnutrition, anaemia, abdominal pain.

Chronic presentations

- Strictures—intermittent colicky abdominal pains associated with eating.
- Malabsorption (due to widespread disease often with previous resections).
- Growth retardation in children (due to chronic malnutrition and chronic inflammatory response suppressing growth).

Extraintestinal features

- Eye: episcleritis, uveitis.
- Acute phase proteins, e.g. C-reactive protein (CRP)
- Joints: arthritis.
- Skin: erythema nodosum, pyoderma gangrenosum.
- Liver: sclerosing cholangitis, cirrhosis.

Perianal disease

Fissure *in ano*, fistula *in ano*, perianal sepsis.

Investigations

- FBC: macrocytic anaemia.
- Acute phase proteins, e.g. C-reactive protein (CRP)
- Small bowel enema: narrowed terminal ileum, 'string sign' of Kantor, stricture formation, fistulae.
- Abdominal ultrasound: RIF mass, abscess formation.
- CT scan: RIF mass, abscess formation.
- Indium-labelled white-cell scan: areas of inflammation.

ESSENTIAL MANAGEMENT

Medical

- Nutritional support (enteral and parenteral feeding).
- Anti-inflammatory drugs (salazopyrin, steroids).
- Antibiotics (only for specific complicating bacterial infections).
- Immunosuppressive agents (azathioprine, cyclosporin A).

Surgical

For

- Complications (peritonitis, obstruction, abscess, fistula).
- Failure of medical treatment and persisting symptoms.
- Growth retardation in children.
- Principles—resect minimum necessary.

Prognosis

- Crohn's disease is a chronic problem, and recurrent episodes of active disease are common.
- 75% of patients will require surgery at some time.
- 60% of patients will require more than one operation.
- Life expectancy of Crohn's disease patients is little different from the 'normal' population.

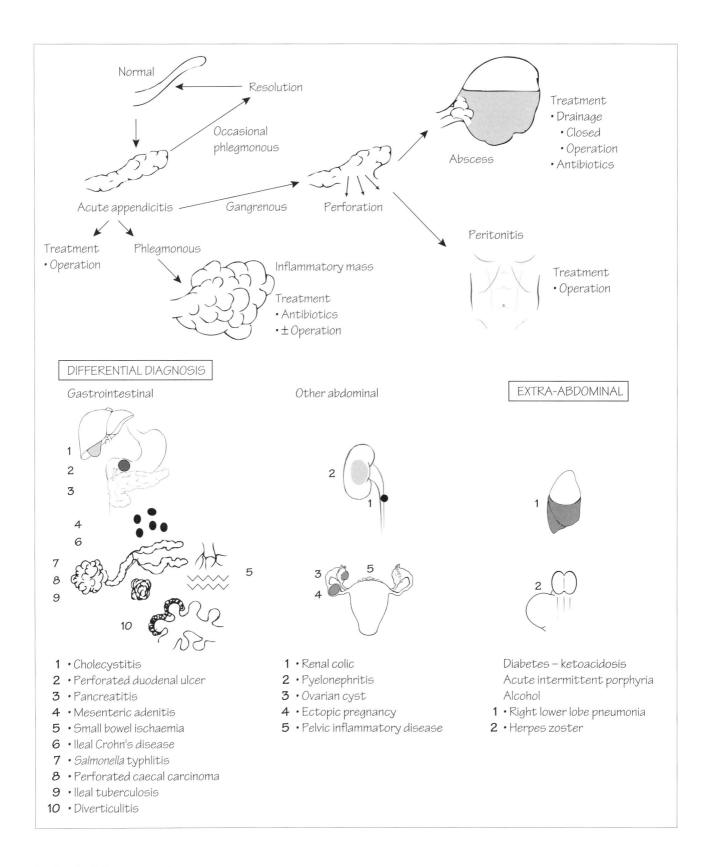

Normal

Resolution

Occasional phlegmonous

Acute appendicitis

Gangrenous

Perforation

Abscess

Treatment
• Drainage
  • Closed
  • Operation
• Antibiotics

Peritonitis

Treatment
• Operation

Treatment
• Operation

Phlegmonous

Inflammatory mass

Treatment
• Antibiotics
• ± Operation

DIFFERENTIAL DIAGNOSIS

Gastrointestinal

Other abdominal

EXTRA-ABDOMINAL

1 • Cholecystitis
2 • Perforated duodenal ulcer
3 • Pancreatitis
4 • Mesenteric adenitis
5 • Small bowel ischaemia
6 • Ileal Crohn's disease
7 • Salmonella typhlitis
8 • Perforated caecal carcinoma
9 • Ileal tuberculosis
10 • Diverticulitis

1 • Renal colic
2 • Pyelonephritis
3 • Ovarian cyst
4 • Ectopic pregnancy
5 • Pelvic inflammatory disease

Diabetes – ketoacidosis
Acute intermittent porphyria
Alcohol
1 • Right lower lobe pneumonia
2 • Herpes zoster

Definition

Acute appendicitis is an inflammation of the vermiform appendix.

Epidemiology

Commonest surgical emergency in the Western world. Rare under 2 years, common in second and third decades, but can occur at any age.

Pathology

- 'Obstructive'—infection superimposed on luminal obstruction from any cause.
- 'Phlegmonous'—viral infection, lymphoid hyperplasia, ulceration, bacterial invasion without obvious cause.

Clinical features

- Periumbilical abdominal pain, nausea, vomiting.
- Localization of pain to RIF.
- Mild pyrexia.
- Patient is flushed, tachycardia, furred tongue, halitosis.
- Tender (usually with rebound) over McBurney's point.
- Right-sided pelvic tenderness on PR examination.
- Peritonitis if appendix perforated.
- Appendix mass if patient presents late.

Investigations

- Diagnosis is a clinical diagnosis, but WCC (almost always leucocytosis) and CRP (usually raised) are helpful.
- Ultrasound for appendix mass and if in doubt to rule out other pelvic pathology (e.g. ovarian cyst).
- Laparoscopy commonly used to exclude ovarian pathology prior to appendicectomy in young women.
- CT scan (helical) in elderly patients or where other causes are considered possible.

Differential diagnosis

- Mesenteric lymphadenitis in children.
- Pelvic disease in women (e.g. pelvic inflammatory disease, UTIs, ectopic pregnancy, ruptured corpus luteum cyst).
- More rarely: Crohn's disease, cholecystitis, perforated duodenal ulcer, right basal pneumonia, torsion of the right testis, diabetes mellitus in younger and middle-aged patients.
- Occasionally: perforated caecal carcinoma, sigmoid diverticulitis, caecal diverticulitis in elderly patients.

ESSENTIAL MANAGEMENT
- Acute appendicitis: appendicectomy, open or laparoscopic.
- Appendix mass: i.v. fluids, antibiotics, close observation. Then:
  If symptoms resolve: interval appendicectomy after a few months.
  If symptoms progress: urgent appendicectomy ± drainage.

Complications

- Wound infection.
- Intra-abdominal abscess (pelvic, RIF, subphrenic).
- Adhesions.
- Abdominal actinomycosis (rare!).
- Portal pyaemia.

43 Diverticular disease

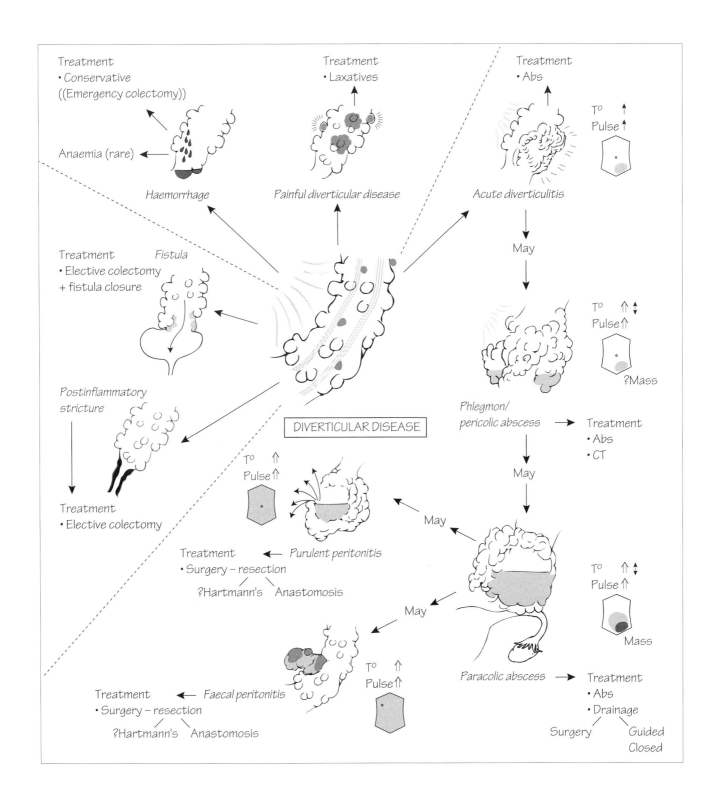

Treatment
• Conservative
((Emergency colectomy))

Anaemia (rare) ←

Haemorrhage

Treatment
• Laxatives

Painful diverticular disease

Treatment
• Abs

Acute diverticulitis

T° ⬆
Pulse ⬆

May

T° ⬆⬍
Pulse ⬆

?Mass

Treatment   *Fistula*
• Elective colectomy
+ fistula closure

*Postinflammatory
stricture*

Treatment
• Elective colectomy

DIVERTICULAR DISEASE

*Phlegmon/
pericolic abscess* → Treatment
• Abs
• CT

May

T° ⬆
Pulse ⬆

Treatment ← *Purulent peritonitis*
• Surgery – resection
?Hartmann's   Anastomosis

May

T° ⬆⬍
Pulse ⬆

Mass

Paracolic abscess → Treatment
• Abs
• Drainage

Surgery   Guided
            Closed

T° ⬆
Pulse ⬆

Treatment ← *Faecal peritonitis*
• Surgery – resection
?Hartmann's   Anastomosis

Definition

Diverticular disease (or diverticulosis) is a condition in which many sac-like mucosal projections (diverticula) develop in the large bowel, especially the sigmoid colon. Acute inflammation of a diverticulum causes diverticulitis.

Epidemiology

Male/female 1 : 1.5, peak incidence 40s and 50s onwards. High incidence in the Western world where it is found in 50% of people over 60 years.

Aetiology

- Low fibre in the diet causes an increase in intraluminal colonic pressure, resulting in herniation of the mucosa through the muscle coats of the wall of the colon.
- Weak areas in wall of colon where nutrient arteries penetrate to submucosa and mucosa.

Pathology

Macroscopic

- Diverticula mostly found in (thickened) sigmoid colon.
- Emerge between the taenia coli and may contain faecoliths.

Histological

Projections are *acquired diverticula* as they contain only mucosa, submucosa and serosa and not all layers of intestinal wall.

Clinical features

- Mostly asymptomatic.
- Painful diverticulosis: LIF pain, constipation, diarrhoea.
- Acute diverticulitis: malaise, fever, LIF pain and tenderness ± palpable mass and abdominal distension.
- Perforation: peritonitis + features of diverticulitis.

- Large bowel obstruction: absolute constipation, distension, colicky abdominal pain and vomiting.
- Fistula: to bladder (cystitis/pneumaturia/recurrent UTIs); to vagina (faecal discharge PV); to small intestine (diarrhoea).
- Lower GI bleed: painless spontaneous—distinguish from angiodysplasia.

Investigations

- Diverticulosis: barium enema (colonoscopy).
- Diverticulitis: FBC, WCC, U+E, chest X-ray, CT scan.
- ?Diverticular mass/paracolic abscess: CT scan.
- ?Perforation: plain film of abdomen, CT scan.
- ?Obstruction: gastrograffin or dilute barium enema, colonoscopy to exclude underlying malignancy.
- ?Fistula:
  colovesical—MSU, cystoscopy, barium enema;
  colovaginal—colposcopy, flexible sigmoidoscopy.
- Haemorrhage: colonoscopy, selective angiography.

ESSENTIAL MANAGEMENT
Medical
Painful or asymptomatic
High-fibre diet (fruit, vegetables, wholemeal breads, bran). Increase fluid intake.

Acute diverticulitis
- Antibiotics and bowel rest.
- Radiologically guided drainage for localized abscess.

Surgical
- Usually for complications/recurrent, proven, acute attacks or (rarely) failed medical treatment.
- Elective left colon surgery without peritonitis: resect diseased colon and rejoin the ends (primary anastomosis).
- Emergency left colon surgery with diffuse peritonitis: resect diseased segment, oversew distal bowel (i.e. upper rectum) and bring out proximal bowel as end-colostomy (Hartmann's procedure).
- Emergency left colon surgery with limited or no peritonitis: resect diseased segment and rejoin the ends (primary anastomosis) may be safe.
- Complicated left colon surgery (e.g. colovesical fistula): resection, primary anastomosis (may have defunctioning proximal stoma).

Prognosis

Diverticular disease is a 'benign' condition, but there is significant mortality and morbidity from the complications.

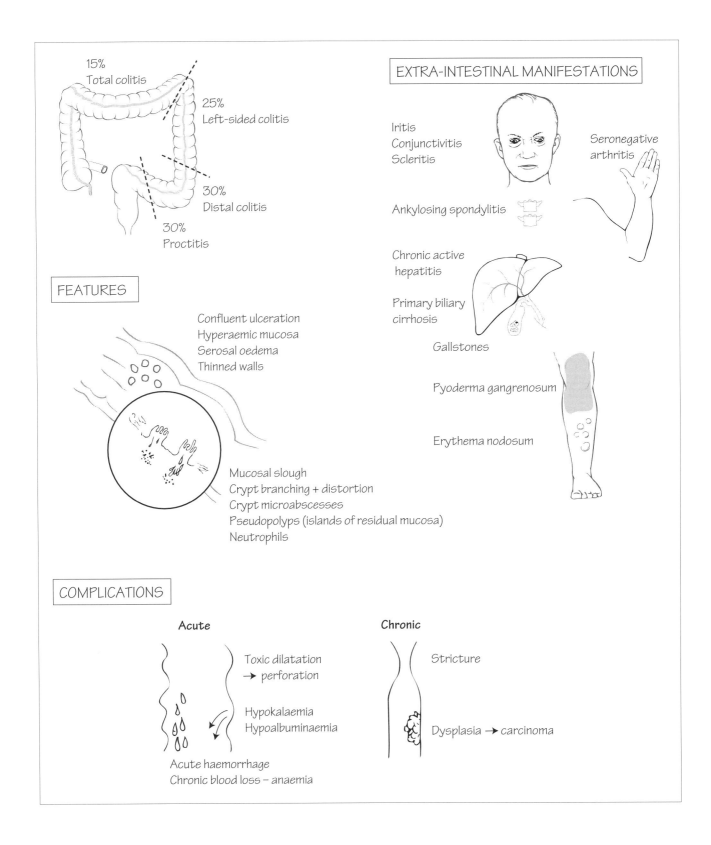

15%
Total colitis

25%
Left-sided colitis

30%
Distal colitis

30%
Proctitis

EXTRA-INTESTINAL MANIFESTATIONS

Iritis
Conjunctivitis
Scleritis

Seronegative
arthritis

Ankylosing spondylitis

Chronic active
 hepatitis

Primary biliary
cirrhosis

Gallstones

Pyoderma gangrenosum

Erythema nodosum

FEATURES

Confluent ulceration
Hyperaemic mucosa
Serosal oedema
Thinned walls

Mucosal slough
Crypt branching + distortion
Crypt microabscesses
Pseudopolyps (islands of residual mucosa)
Neutrophils

COMPLICATIONS

Acute

Toxic dilatation
→ perforation

Hypokalaemia
Hypoalbuminaemia

Acute haemorrhage
Chronic blood loss – anaemia

Chronic

Stricture

Dysplasia → carcinoma

Definition

A chronic inflammatory disorder of the colonic mucosa, usually beginning in the rectum and extending proximally to a variable extent.

> **KEY POINTS**
> - The majority of colitis is controlled by medical management—surgery is usually only required for poor control of symptoms or complications.
> - Acute attacks require close scrutiny to avoid major complications.
> - Long-term colitis carries a risk of colonic malignancy.
> - Ileoanal pouch reconstruction offers good function in the majority of cases where surgery is required.

Epidemiology

Male/female 1 : 1.6, peak incidence 30–50 years. High incidence among relatives of patients (up to 40%) and among Europeans and Jewish people.

Aetiology

- Genetic origin: increased prevalence (10%) in relatives, associated with HLA-B27 phenotype.
- May have autoimmune basis.
- Smoking protects against relapse!

Pathology

Disease confined to colon, rectum always involved, may be 'backwash' ileitis.

Macroscopic

Only the mucosa is involved with superficial ulceration, exudation and pseudopolyposis.

Histological

Crypt abscess, inflammatory polyps and highly vascular granulation tissue. Epithelial dysplasia with longstanding disease.

Clinical features

Proctitis

- Mucus, pus and blood PR.
- Diarrhoea with urgency and frequency.

Left-sided colitis → total colitis

Symptoms of proctitis + increasing features of systemic upset, abdominal pain, anorexia, weight loss and anaemia with more extensive disease.

Extraintestinal features

Percentage involved:
- joints: arthritis (25%);
- eye: uveitis (10%);
- skin: erythema nodosum, pyoderma gangrenosum (10%);
- liver: pericholangitis, fatty liver (3%);
- blood: thromboembolic disease (rare).

Severe/fulminant disease

- 6–20 bloody bowel motions per day.
- Fever, anaemia, dehydration, electrolyte imbalance.
- Colonic dilatation/perforation—'toxic megacolon'.

Investigations

- FBC: iron deficiency anaemia.
- Stool culture: exclude infective colitis before treatment.
- Plain abdominal radiograph: colonic dilatation or air under diaphragm indicating perforation in fulminant colitis.
- Barium enema: loss of haustrations, shortened lead pipe colon.
- Sigmoidoscopy: inflamed friable mucosa, bleeds to touch.
- Colonoscopy: extent of disease at presentation, evaluation of response to treatment after exacerbations, screening of long-standing disease for dysplasia.
- Biopsy: typical histological features.

ESSENTIAL MANAGEMENT

Medical
- Basic: high-fibre diet, antidiarrhoeal agents (codeine phosphate, loperamide).
- First-line: anti-inflammatory drugs (salazopyrin, 5 aminosalicylic acid (5-ASA), corticosteroids).
- Second-line: other immunosuppressive agents (azathioprine, cyclosporin A).
- Use enemas if disease confined to rectum.
- Oral preparations for more extensive disease.
- i.v. immunosuppressives for acute exacerbations.

Surgical

Indications
- Failure of medical treatment to control chronic symptoms.
- Complications: profuse haemorrhage, perforation/toxic megacolon, risk of cancer (greater with longer disease, more aggressive onset and more extensive disease).
- Dysplasia or development of carcinoma

Operations
- For acute attacks/complications—total colectomy, end ileostomy and preserved rectal stump.
- Electively—proctocolectomy with end (Brooke) ileostomy *or* proctocolectomy with preservation of anal sphincter and creation of ileoanal pouch (e.g. J-shaped pouch).

Prognosis

Ulcerative colitis is a chronic problem that requires constant surveillance unless surgery, which is drastic but curative, is performed.

45 Colorectal carcinoma

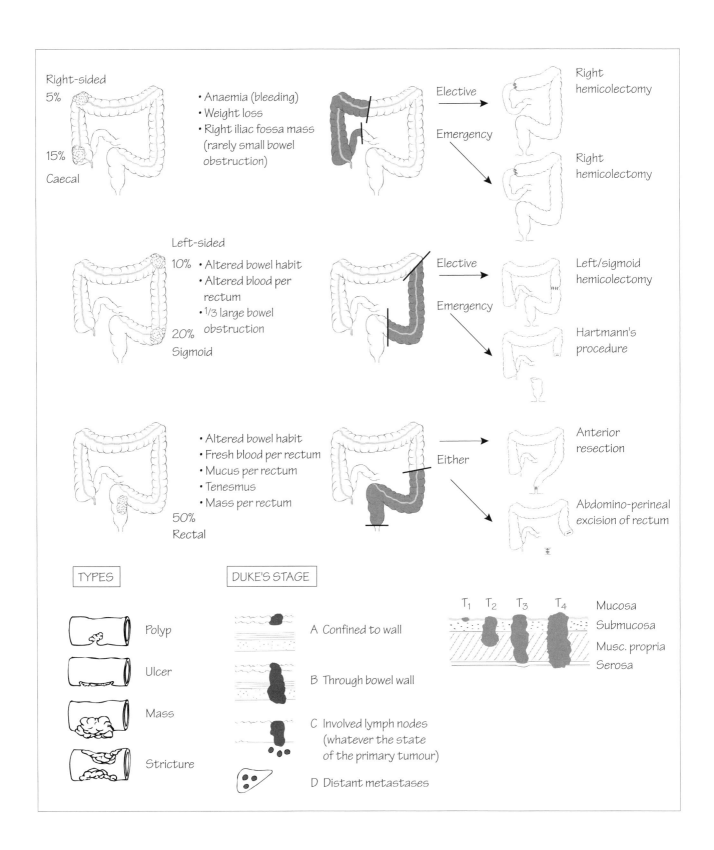

Definition

Colorectal carcinoma (CRC) is the occurrence of malignant lesions in the mucosa of the colon or rectum.

KEY POINTS

- Genetic factors play an important role in risk of CRC.
- Most colorectal cancers are left sided and produce symptoms of bleeding or altered bowel habit.
- Prognosis depends mainly on stage at diagnosis.
- Surgery is the only curative treatment but radiotherapy and chemotherapy are both useful adjuncts.

Epidemiology

Male/female 1.3 : 1, peak incidence 50+ years. Incidence has increased in Western world over last 50 years.

Aetiology

Predisposing factors in decreasing importance:

- a prior CRC or adenomatous polyps;
- hereditary polyposis syndromes;
- family history of CRC; or
- chronic active ulcerative colitis;
- diet (low in indigestible fibre, high in animal fat);
- increased faecal bile salts, selenium deficiency.

Pathology

Macroscopic

- Polypoid, ulcerating, annular, infiltrative.
- 75% of lesions are within 60 cm of the anal margin (rectum, sigmoid, left colon).
- 3% are synchronous (i.e. a second lesion will be found at the same time) and 3% are metachronous (i.e. a second lesion will be found later).

Histological

- Adenocarcinoma (10–15% are mucinous adenocarcinoma).
- Staging by Dukes' classification and TNM.
- Spread: lymphatic, haematogenous (via veins to liver), peritoneal.

Clinical features

- Anaemia—caecal cancers often present with anaemia.
- Colicky abdominal pain—tumours which are causing partial obstruction, e.g. transverse or descending colonic lesions.
- Alteration in bowel habit—either constipation or diarrhoea.

- Bleeding or passage of mucus PR.
- Tenesmus (frequent or continuous desire to defaecate)—rectal lesions.

Investigations

- Digital rectal examination and faecal occult blood.
- FBC: anaemia.
- U+E: hypokalaemia, LFTs: liver metastases.
- Sigmoidoscopy (rigid to 30 cm/flexible to 60 cm) and colonoscopy (whole colon)—see the lesion, obtain biopsy.
- Double-contrast barium enema—'apple core lesion', polyp.
- CEA is often raised in advanced disease.

ESSENTIAL MANAGEMENT

Surgery (potentially curative)

Resection of the tumour with adequate margins to include regional lymph nodes.

Procedures

- Right hemicolectomy (no bowel preparation) for lesions from caecum to splenic flexure.
- Left hemicolectomy (bowel preparation) for lesions of descending and sigmoid colon.
- Anterior resection for rectal tumours.
- Abdomino-perineal resection and colostomy for very low rectal lesions.
- Hartmann's procedure for emergency surgery to left colon.
- Resection possible for liver metastases if fewer than five are present.

Surgery/interventions (palliative)

- Open resection of the tumour (with anastomosis or stoma) for obstructing or symptomatic cancers despite metastases.
- Surgical bypass for obstructing inoperable cancers.
- Transanal resection for inoperable rectal cancer.
- Intraluminal stents for obstructing cancers.

Other treatment

- Radiotherapy may be used to shrink rectal cancers preoperatively or palliate inoperable rectal cancer.
- Adjuvant chemotherapy (5-FU ± levamisole) to reduce risk of systemic recurrence (Dukes' C and some Dukes' B) or palliate liver metastases.

Prognosis

- 5-year survival depends on staging: A, 80%; B, 60%; C, 35%; D, 5%.
- 25% 5-year survival after successful resections of <5 liver metastases.

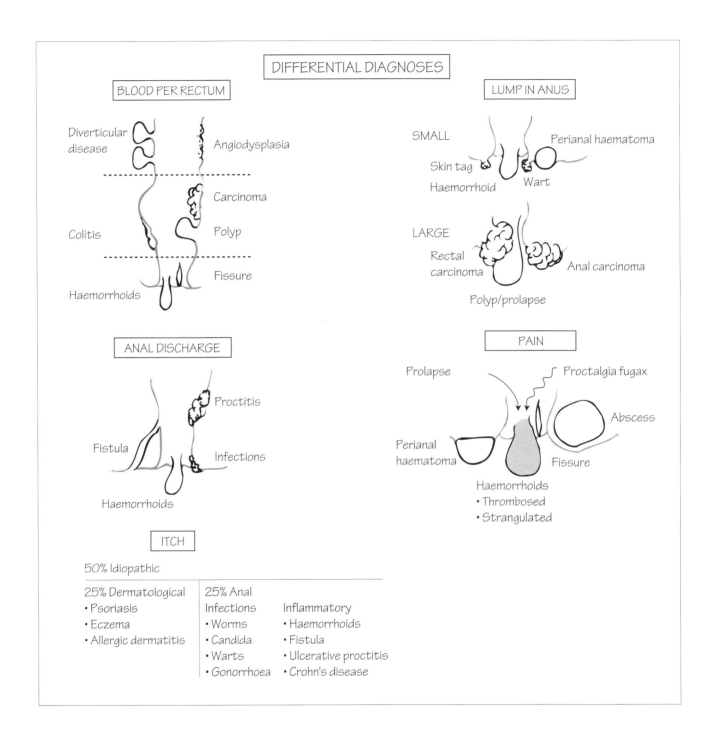

DIFFERENTIAL DIAGNOSES

BLOOD PER RECTUM

Diverticular disease

Angiodysplasia

Carcinoma

Colitis

Polyp

Fissure

Haemorrhoids

LUMP IN ANUS

SMALL

Skin tag

Perianal haematoma

Haemorrhoid

Wart

LARGE

Rectal carcinoma

Anal carcinoma

Polyp/prolapse

ANAL DISCHARGE

Proctitis

Fistula

Infections

Haemorrhoids

PAIN

Prolapse

Proctalgia fugax

Abscess

Perianal haematoma

Fissure

Haemorrhoids
• Thrombosed
• Strangulated

ITCH

50% Idiopathic

25% Dermatological	25% Anal Infections	Inflammatory
• Psoriasis	• Worms	• Haemorrhoids
• Eczema	• Candida	• Fistula
• Allergic dermatitis	• Warts	• Ulcerative proctitis
	• Gonorrhoea	• Crohn's disease

Haemorrhoids ('piles')

Definition

A submucosal swelling in the anal canal consisting of a dilated venous plexus, a small artery and areolar tissue. Internal: only involves tissue of upper anal canal. External: involves tissue of lower anal canal.

Aetiology

• Increased venous pressure from straining (low-fibre diet) or altered haemodynamics (e.g. during pregnancy) causes chronic dilation of submucosal venous plexus.
• Found at the 3, 7 and 11 o'clock positions in the anal canal.

Clinical features
- First degree (1°): bleeding/itching only.
- Second degree (2°): prolapse during defaecation.
- Third degree (3°): constantly prolapsed.

Treatment
- Simple treatment—bulk laxatives and high-fibre diet.
- Bleeding internal piles—injection sclerotherapy, Barron's bands, cryosurgery.
- Prolapsing external—haemorrhoidectomy (complications: bleeding, anal stenosis).

Rectal prolapse
Definition
The protrusion from the anus to a variable degree of the rectal mucosa (partial) or rectal wall (full thickness).

Aetiology
Rectal intussusception, poor sphincter tone, chronic straining, pelvic floor injury.

Clinical features
Mucous discharge, bleeding, tenesmus, obvious prolapse.

Treatment
Stool manipulation and biofeedback, Delorme's perianal mucosal resection, abdominal rectopexy (rectum is 'hitched' up onto sacrum).

Perianal haematoma
Very painful subcutaneous haematoma caused by rupture of small blood vessel in the perianal area. Evacuation of the clot provides instant relief.

Anal fissure
Definition
Longitudinal tear in the mucosa of the anal canal, in the midline posteriorly (90%) or anteriorly (10%).

Aetiology
- 90% caused by local trauma during passage of constipated stool and potentiated by spasm of the internal anal sphincter.
- Other causes: pregnancy/delivery, Crohn's disease, sexually transmitted infections (often lateral position).

Clinical features
Exquisitely painful on passing bowel motion, small amount of bright red blood on toilet tissue, severe sphincter spasm, skin tag at distal end of tear ('sentinel pile').

Treatment
- First-line: stool softeners/bulking agents, local anaesthetic (LA) gels, GTN ointment.
- Second-line: botulinum toxin injection, lateral internal sphincterotomy.
- Examination under anaesthesia (EUA) and biopsy for atypical/suspicious abnormal fissures.

Perianal abscess
Aetiology
Focus of infection starts in anal glands ('cryptoglandular sepsis') and spreads into perianal tissues to cause:
- perianal abscess: adjacent to anal margin;
- ischiorectal abscess: in ischiorectal fossa;
- para-rectal abscess: above levator ani.

Clinical features
Painful, red, tender, swollen mass ± fever, rigors, sweating, tachycardia.

Treatment
Incision and drainage, antibiotics.

Fistula *in ano*
Definition and aetiology
Abnormal communication between the perianal skin and the anal canal, established and persisting following drainage of a perianal abscess. May be associated with Crohn's disease (multiple fistulae), UC or TB.
- Low: below 50% of the external anal sphincter (EAS).
- High: crossing 50% or more of the EAS.

Clinical features
Chronic perianal discharge, external orifice of track with granulation tissue seen perianally.

Treatment
- Low: probing and laying open the track (fistulotomy).
- High: seton insertion, core removal of the fistula track.

Pilonidal sinus
Definition
A blind-ending track containing hairs in the skin of the natal cleft.

Aetiology
Movement of buttocks promotes hair migration into a (?congenital) sinus.

Clinical features
May present as: a natal cleft abscess, a discharging sinus in midline posterior to anal margin with hair protruding from orifice, natal cleft itch/pain.

Treatment
Good personal hygiene. Incision and drainage of abscesses, excision of sinus network.

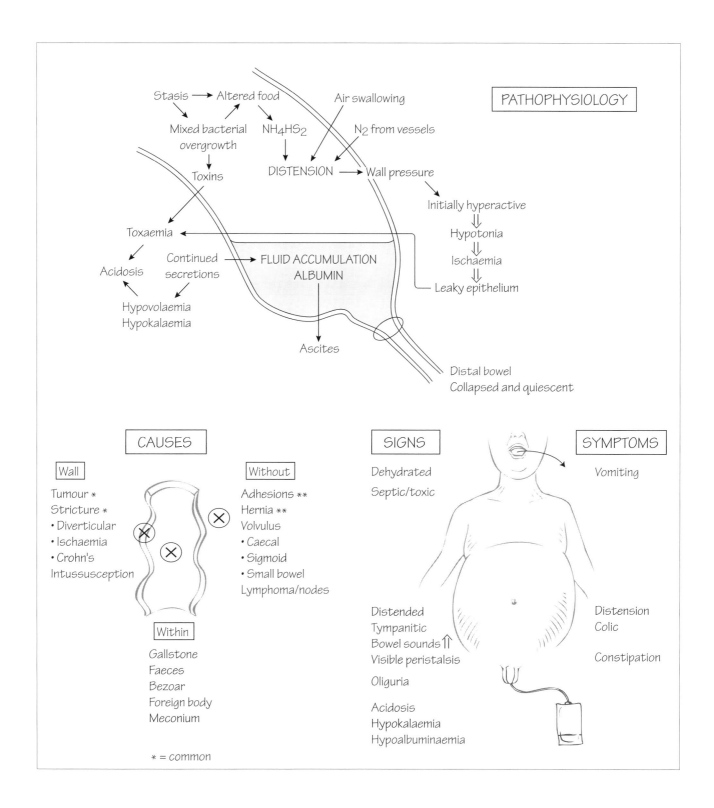

PATHOPHYSIOLOGY

Stasis → Altered food   Air swallowing

Mixed bacterial   NH₄HS₂   N₂ from vessels
overgrowth

Toxins   DISTENSION → Wall pressure

Initially hyperactive

Toxaemia   Hypotonia

Acidosis   Continued   FLUID ACCUMULATION   Ischaemia
secretions   ALBUMIN
Leaky epithelium

Hypovolaemia
Hypokalaemia

Ascites

Distal bowel
Collapsed and quiescent

CAUSES   SIGNS   SYMPTOMS

Wall   Without   Dehydrated   Vomiting
Tumour *   Adhesions **   Septic/toxic
Stricture *   Hernia **
• Diverticular   Volvulus
• Ischaemia   • Caecal
• Crohn's   • Sigmoid
Intussusception   • Small bowel
Lymphoma/nodes

Distended   Distension
Tympanitic   Colic
Within   Bowel sounds ⇑
Gallstone   Visible peristalsis   Constipation
Faeces   Oliguria
Bezoar
Foreign body   Acidosis
Meconium   Hypokalaemia
Hypoalbuminaemia

* = common

Definitions

Complete intestinal obstruction indicates total blockage of the intestinal lumen, whereas *incomplete* denotes only a partial blockage. Obstruction may be *acute* (hours) or *chronic* (weeks), *simple* (*mechanical*), i.e. blood supply is not compromised, or *strangulated*, i.e. blood supply is compromised. A *closed loop obstruction* indicates that both the inlet and outlet of a bowel loop is closed off.

KEY POINTS

- Small bowel obstruction is often rapid in onset and commonly due to adhesions or hernia.
- Large bowel obstruction may be gradual or intermittent in onset, is often due to carcinoma or strictures and NEVER due to adhesions.
- All obstructed patients need fluid and electrolyte replacement.
- The cause should be sought and confirmed wherever possible prior to operation.
- Tachycardia, pyrexia and abdominal tenderness indicate the need to operate whatever the cause.

Common causes

- Extramural: adhesions, bands, volvulus, hernias (internal and external), compression by tumour (e.g. frozen pelvis).
- Intramural: inflammatory bowel disease (Crohn's disease), tumours, carcinomas, lymphomas, strictures, paralytic: (adynamic) ileus, intussusception.
- Intraluminal: faecal impaction, foreign bodies, bezoars, gallstone ileus.

Pathophysiology

- Bowel distal to obstruction collapses.
- Bowel proximal to obstruction distends and becomes hyperactive. Distension is due to swallowed air and accumulating intestinal secretions.
- The bowel wall becomes oedematous. Fluid and electrolytes accumulate in the wall and lumen (third space loss).
- Bacteria proliferate in the obstructed bowel.
- As the bowel distends, the intramural vessels become stretched and the blood supply is compromised, leading to ischaemia and necrosis.

Clinical features

- Vomiting, colicky abdominal pain, abdominal distension, absolute constipation (i.e. neither faeces nor flatus).
- Dehydration and loss of skin turgor.
- Hypotension, tachycardia.
- Abdominal distension and increased bowel sounds.
- Empty rectum on digital examination.
- Tenderness or rebound indicates peritonitis.

Investigations

- Hb, PCV: elevated due to dehydration.
- WCC: normal or slightly elevated.
- U+E: urea elevated, Na^+ and Cl^- low.
- Chest X-ray: elevated diaphragm due to abdominal distension.
- Abdominal supine X-ray:
  (a) small bowel (central loops, non-anatomical distribution, valvulae conniventes shadows cross entire width of lumen) or large bowel obstruction (peripheral distribution/haustral shadows do not cross entire width of bowel).
  (b) look for cause (gallstone, characteristic patterns of volvulus, hernias).
- Single contrast large bowel enema—?large bowel obstruction—site and cause.
- CT scan—?small bowel obstruction—site and cause, sigmoidoscopy to show site of obstruction.

ESSENTIAL MANAGEMENT

- Decompress the obstructed gut: pass nasogastric tube.
- Replace fluid and electrolyte losses: give Ringer's lactate or NaCl with K^+ supplementation.
- Monitor the patient—fluid balance chart, urinary catheter, regular temperature, pulse, respiration (TPR) chart, blood tests.
- Request investigations appropriate to likely cause.
  - Relieve the obstruction surgically if:
  - underlying causes need surgical treatment (e.g. hernia, colonic carcinoma);
  - patient does not improve with conservative treatment (e.g. adhesion obstruction); or
  - there are signs of strangulation or peritonitis.

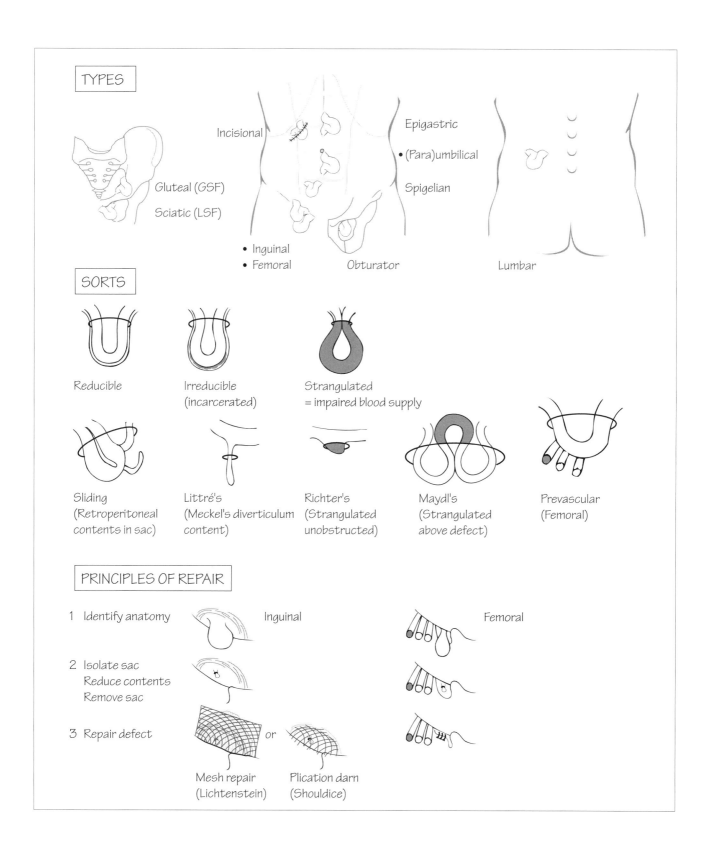

TYPES

Incisional

Gluteal (GSF)

Sciatic (LSF)

Epigastric

• (Para)umbilical

Spigelian

• Inguinal
• Femoral

Obturator

Lumbar

SORTS

Reducible

Irreducible
(incarcerated)

Strangulated
= impaired blood supply

Sliding
(Retroperitoneal
contents in sac)

Littré's
(Meckel's diverticulum
content)

Richter's
(Strangulated
unobstructed)

Maydl's
(Strangulated
above defect)

Prevascular
(Femoral)

PRINCIPLES OF REPAIR

1 Identify anatomy

Inguinal

Femoral

2 Isolate sac
   Reduce contents
   Remove sac

3 Repair defect

Mesh repair
(Lichtenstein)

or

Plication darn
(Shouldice)

Definition

A hernia is the protrusion of a viscus or part of a viscus through an abnormal opening in its coverings.

Types

Common

- Umbilical/para-umbilical.
- Inguinal (direct and indirect).
- Femoral.
- Incisional.

Uncommon

- Epigastric.
- Gluteal, lumbar, obturator.

Pathophysiology

- The defect in the abdominal wall may be congenital (e.g. umbilical hernia, femoral canal) or acquired (e.g. an incision) and is lined with peritoneum (the sac).
- Raised intra-abdominal pressure further weakens the defect allowing some of the intra-abdominal contents (e.g. omentum, small bowel loop) to migrate through the opening.
- Entrapment of the contents in the sac leads to incarceration (unable to reduce contents) and possibly strangulation (blood supply to incarcerated contents is compromised).

Clinical features

- Patient presents with a lump over the site of the hernia.
- Femoral hernias are below and lateral to the pubic tubercle, they usually flatten the groin crease and are 10 times more common in women than men. 50% present as a surgical emergency due to obstructed contents and 50% of these will require a small bowel resection. Femoral hernias are irreducible.

- Inguinal hernias start off above and medial to the pubic tubercle but may descend broadly when larger, they usually accentuate the groin crease. Most are benign and have a low risk of complications.

  (a) Indirect inguinal hernias can be controlled by digital pressure over the internal inguinal ring, may be narrow necked and are common in younger men (3% per annum present with complications).

  (b) Direct inguinal hernias are poorly controlled by digital pressure, are often broad necked and are commoner in older men (0.3% per annum strangulate).

- Incisional hernias bulge, are usually broad necked, poorly controlled by pressure and are accentuated by tensing the recti. Large, chronic incisional hernias may contain much of the small bowel and may by irreducible/unrepairable due to the 'loss of the right of abode in the abdomen' of the contents.
- True umbilical hernias are present from birth and are symmetrical defects in the umbilicus due to failure to close.
- Para-umbilical hernias develop due to an acquired defect in the periumbilical fascia.

Complications of surgery

- Haematoma (wound or scrotal).
- Acute urinary retention.
- Wound infection.
- Chronic pain.
- Testicular pain and swelling leading to testicular atrophy.
- Hernia recurrence (about 5%).

	Causes and symptoms	Cardinal symptoms and signs	Structure involved (diagnosis)		
			Gallbladder	CBD	Other
A	Presence of stone → Irritation → Contraction	Pain Nausea Vomiting Tender RUQ	Biliary colic ⋮ May ↓	Biliary (ductal) colic ⋮ May	—
B	Obstruction of structure (simple)	As above + • Persistence of pain etc. • Mass RUQ (jaundice)	Mucocele ⋮ May ↓	Obstructive jaundice ⋮ May	—
C	Obstruction of structure (+ infection)	As above + • Swinging fever • Tachycardia • Neutrophilia • Rigors	Empyema ⋮ May ↓ perforate Biliary peritonitis	Cholangitis	—
D	Inflammation/ infection	As for A + • Fever • Tachycardia • Neutrophilia	Cholecystitis	(Cholangitis)	Pancreatitis

Other conditions associated with gallstones
• Gallstone ileus
• Adenocarcinoma gallbladder

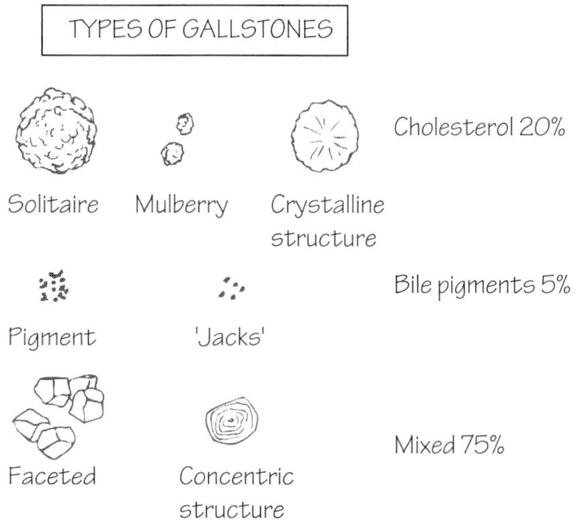

CAUSES

TYPES OF GALLSTONES

Solitaire   Mulberry   Crystalline structure

Cholesterol 20%

Pigment   'Jacks'

Bile pigments 5%

Faceted   Concentric structure

Mixed 75%

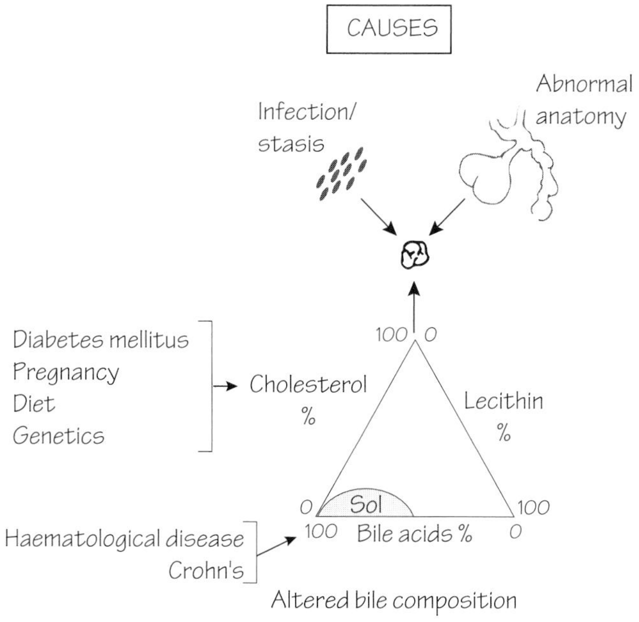

Infection/ stasis

Abnormal anatomy

Diabetes mellitus
Pregnancy
Diet
Genetics
→ Cholesterol %

Lecithin %

Sol

Haematological disease
Crohn's
→ Bile acids %

Altered bile composition

Definition

Gallstones are round, oval or faceted concretions found in the biliary tract. They contain cholesterol, calcium carbonate, calcium bilirubinate or a mixture of these elements.

Epidemiology

Male/female 1 : 2. Age 40s onwards. High incidence of mixed stones in Western world. Pigment stones commoner in the East.

Pathogenesis

- Cholesterol stones: imbalance in bile between cholesterol, bile salts and phospholipids, producing lithogenic bile. Associated with inflammatory bowel disease.
- Bilirubinate stones: chronic haemolysis, infection with α-glucuronidase-producing bacteria.
- Mixed stones: associated with anatomical abnormalities, stasis, previous surgery, previous infections.

Pathology

- Gallstones passing through the biliary system may cause biliary colic or pancreatitis.
- Stone obstruction at the gallbladder neck with superimposed infection leads to cholecystitis.
- Obstruction of the common bile duct (CBD) with superimposed infection leads to septic cholangitis.
- Migration of a large stone into the gut may cause intestinal obstruction (gallstone ileus).

Clinical features

- 90% of gallstones are (probably) asymptomatic.
- Biliary colic: severe colicky upper abdominal pain radiating around the right costal margin ± vomiting. Periodicity of hours, often onset at night spontaneously resolves after several hours. Differential diagnosis includes myocardial infarction, peptic ulcer exacerbation, GORD.
- 'Chronic cholecystitis': uncertain diagnosis suggested by vague, intermittent right upper abdominal pain, distension, flatulence, fatty food intolerance. May indicate recurrent mild episodes of cholecystitis. Differential diagnosis includes chronic PUD, GORD.
- Acute obstructive cholecystitis: constant right hypochondrial pain, pyrexia, nausea ± jaundice. Tender in RUQ with positive Murphy's sign. Leucocytosis. Unresolved may lead to an empyema of the gallbladder. Differential diagnosis includes myocardial infarction, basal pneumonia, pancreatitis, appendicitis, perforated peptic ulcer, pulmonary embolus.
- Cholangitis: abdominal pain, high fever/rigors, obstructive jaundice (Charcot's triad), severe RUQ tenderness. Differential diagnosis includes myocardial infarction, basal pneumonia, pancreatitis, acute hepatitis.
- Obstructive jaundice: upper abdominal pain, pale/claylike stools, dark brown urine, pruritus. May progress into cholangitis if CBD remains obstructed.
- Pancreatitis (see p. 114): central/epigastric pain, back pain, fever, tachycardia, epigastric tenderness.

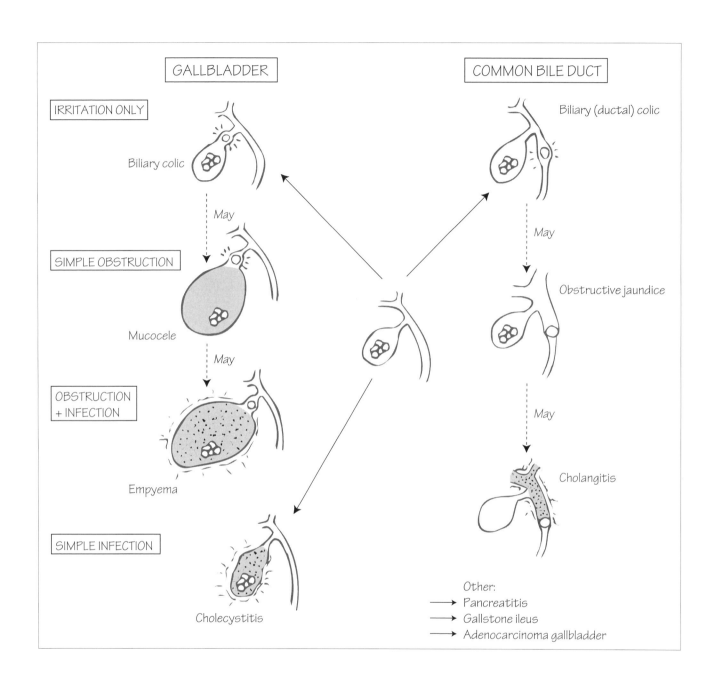

Investigations

• FBC: acute inflammatory complications, picture of haemolytic anaemias underlying.

• U+E.

• LFTs: obstructive jaundice pattern.

• Plain X-ray of the abdomen shows only 10% of gallstones.

• Ultrasound: 90% of gallstones will be detected on ultrasound examination. Assesses CBD size and possible presence of CBD stones.

• Rarely are other investigations, such as oral cholecystography, intravenous cholangiography or HIDA scanning, required (ultrasound impossible, e.g. obesity).

• Endoscopic retrograde cholangiopancreatography (ERCP)—suspected or proven CBD stones. Allows stones removal or stent to be placed to bypass any risk of obstruction from the stones.

• OGD: to exclude PUD as a cause for uncomplicated disease symptoms.

ESSENTIAL MANAGEMENT

• Asymptomatic: no treatment required unless diabetic or undergoing major immunosuppression (risk factors for cholecystitis).

• Biliary colic: elective cholecystectomy, now usually performed laparoscopically, for classic symptoms with ultrasound-proven gallstones.

• Chronic cholecystitis: elective laparoscopic cholecystectomy only if no evidence of PUD or other causes for symptoms.

• Acute cholecystitis: i.v. fluids, antibiotics, early or interval cholecystectomy.

• Empyema: percutaneous (ultrasound- or CT-guided) drainage of the gallbladder and interval cholecystectomy.

• Ascending cholangitis: i.v. fluids, antibiotics, ductal drainage (now usually by ERCP, sphincterotomy and extraction of stones).

Complications of cholecystectomy

• Leakage of bile from cystic duct or gallbladder bed.

• Jaundice due to retained ductal stones. (Retained stones can be treated by ERCP or if a T-tube is in place by extraction with a Dormia basket down the T-tube track (Burhenne manoeuvre).)

• Injury to the CBD.

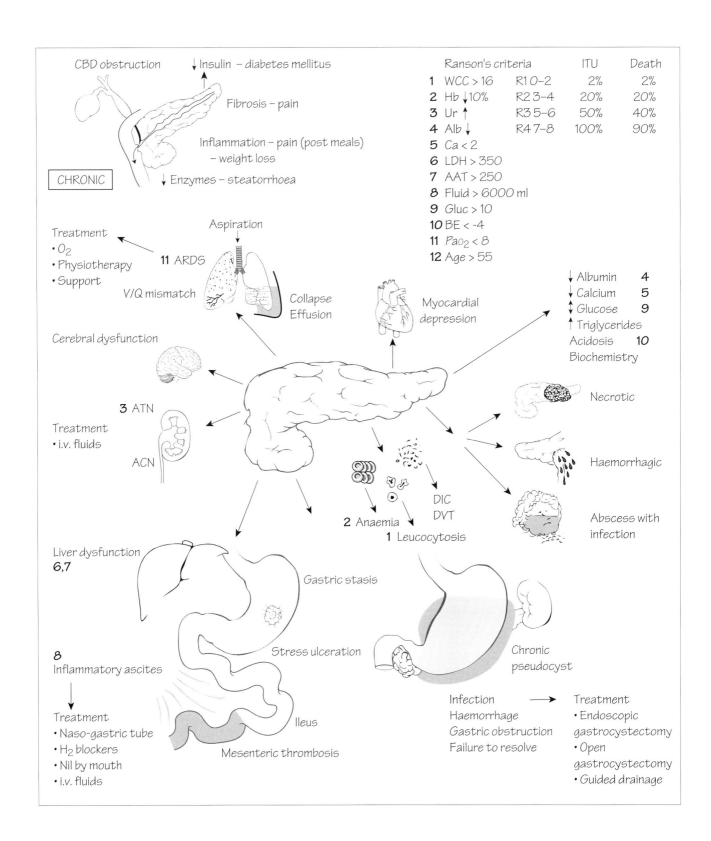

CBD obstruction

↓ Insulin – diabetes mellitus

Fibrosis – pain

Inflammation – pain (post meals)
– weight loss

CHRONIC

↓ Enzymes – steatorrhoea

Ranson's criteria		ITU	Death
1 WCC > 16	R1 0–2	2%	2%
2 Hb ↓10%	R2 3–4	20%	20%
3 Ur ↑	R3 5–6	50%	40%
4 Alb ↓	R4 7–8	100%	90%
5 Ca < 2			
6 LDH > 350			
7 AAT > 250			
8 Fluid > 6000 ml			
9 Gluc > 10			
10 BE < -4			
11 Pao_2 < 8			
12 Age > 55			

Treatment
• O_2
• Physiotherapy
• Support

11 ARDS

Aspiration

V/Q mismatch

Collapse
Effusion

Myocardial
depression

↓ Albumin   4
↓ Calcium   5
↕ Glucose   9
↑ Triglycerides
Acidosis   10
Biochemistry

Cerebral dysfunction

3 ATN

Treatment
• i.v. fluids

ACN

Necrotic

Haemorrhagic

DIC
DVT

2 Anaemia

1 Leucocytosis

Abscess with
infection

Liver dysfunction
6,7

Gastric stasis

8
Inflammatory ascites

Stress ulceration

Treatment
• Naso-gastric tube
• H_2 blockers
• Nil by mouth
• i.v. fluids

Ileus

Mesenteric thrombosis

Chronic
pseudocyst

Infection ⟶ Treatment
Haemorrhage • Endoscopic
Gastric obstruction   gastrocystectomy
Failure to resolve • Open
                     gastrocystectomy
                   • Guided drainage

Definition

An inflammatory condition of the exocrine pancreas that results from injury to the acinar cells. It may be acute or chronic.

> **KEY POINTS**
> - Most pancreatitis is mild and spontaneously resolves.
> - All patients should have a cause sought by imaging and the severity assessed by recognized criteria.
> - A normal or mildly elevated serum amylase does NOT exclude pancreatitis.
> - Severe or complicated pancreatitis may worsen rapidly and require ICU support.
> - Surgery has little place other than to treat severe complications.

Aetiology

- Gallstones and alcohol abuse account for 95% of cases of acute pancreatitis.
- Other causes include: idiopathic, congenital structural abnormalities, drugs, viral infections, hypercalcaemia, hypothermia, hyperlipidaemia and trauma.

Pathology

Acute

- Mild injury: acinar(exocrine) cell damage with enzymatic spillage, inflammatory cascade activation and localized oedema. Local exudate may also lead to increased serum levels of pancreatic enzymes (amylase, lipase, colipase).
- Moderate injury: increasing local inflammation leads to intrapancreatic bleeding, fluid collections and spreading local oedema involving the mesentery and retroperitoneum. Activation of the systemic inflammatory response leads to progressive involvement of other organs.
- Severe injury: progressive pancreatic destruction leads to necrosis, profound localized bleeding and fluid collections around the pancreas. Spread to local structures and the peritoneal cavity may result in mesenteric infarction, peritonitis and intra-abdominal fat 'saponification'.

A persisting accumulation of inflammatory fluid, usually in the lesser sac, is a pseudocyst, i.e. does not have an epithelial lining.

Chronic

Recurrent episodes of acute inflammation lead to progressive destruction of acinar cells with healing by fibrosis. Incidental islet cell damage may lead to endocrine gland failure.

Clinical features

- Mild/moderate pancreatitis: constant upper abdominal pain radiating to back, nausea, vomiting, pyrexia, tachycardia ± jaundice.
- Severe/necrotizing pancreatitis: severe upper abdominal pain, signs of hypovolaemic shock, respiratory and renal impairment, silent abdomen, retroperitoneal bleeding with flank and umbilical bruising (Grey Turner's and Cullen's signs).

> **ESSENTIAL MANAGEMENT**
> - Attempt to confirm diagnosis: (serum amylase > 1000 iμ diagnostic—may be clinical diagnosis).
> - Assess disease severity (Imrie/Ranson criteria).
>   Severe is 3+ of the following: WBC >16 × 10^9/l, Pao_2 <7.98 kPa, B glucose > 11.2 mmol/l, LDH >350 IU/l, SGOT > 250 IU/l, PCV fall > 10%, urea > 1.8, Ca^{2+} < 2.0 mmol/l.
> - Resuscitate the patient:
>   Mild/moderate disease: i.v. fluids, analgesia, monitor progress with pulse, BP, temperature.
>   Severe pancreatitis: full resuscitation in ICU with invasive monitoring.
> - Establish the cause: ultrasound to look for gallstones.
>
> **Further management**
> - No proven use for routine nasogastric tube or antibiotics.
> - ?Vitamin supplements and sedatives if alcoholic cause.
> - Proven CBD gallstones may require urgent ERCP.
> - Failure to respond to treatment or uncertain diagnosis warrants abdominal CT scan.
> - Suspected/proven infection of necrotic pancreas—antibiotics ± surgical debridement.

Complications—acute pancreatitis

Acute

- Pancreatic abscess: usually necrotic pancreas present.
- Intra-abdominal sepsis.
- Necrosis of the transverse colon.
- Respiratory (ARDS) or renal (ATN) failure.
- Pancreatic haemorrhage.

Subacute/chronic

- Pseudocyst formation: may need to be drained internally or externally.
- Chronic pancreatitis.

Chronic pancreatitis

- Usually caused by chronic alcohol abuse.
- Presents with intractable abdominal pain and evidence of exocrine pancreatic failure (steatorrhoea) and eventually diabetes as well.
- Medical treatment is with analgesia and exocrine pancreatic enzyme replacement. Surgical treatment is by drainage of dilated pancreatic ducts or excision of the pancreas in some cases.

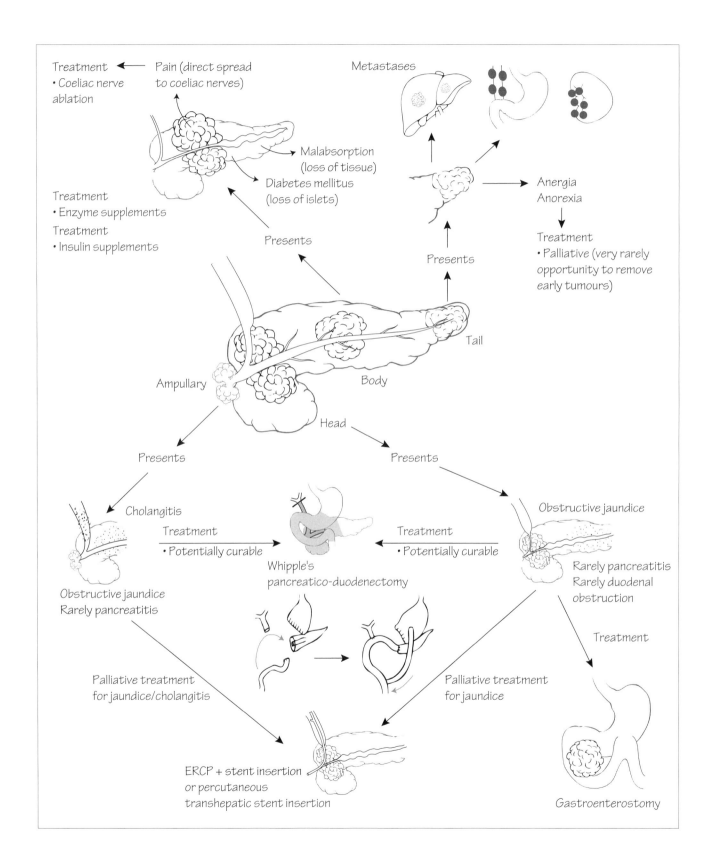

Treatment
• Coeliac nerve ablation

Pain (direct spread to coeliac nerves)

Metastases

Malabsorption (loss of tissue)
Diabetes mellitus (loss of islets)

Treatment
• Enzyme supplements
Treatment
• Insulin supplements

Anergia
Anorexia

Treatment
• Palliative (very rarely opportunity to remove early tumours)

Presents

Presents

Presents

Tail

Ampullary

Body

Head

Presents

Presents

Cholangitis

Obstructive jaundice

Treatment
• Potentially curable

Treatment
• Potentially curable

Whipple's pancreatico-duodenectomy

Rarely pancreatitis
Rarely duodenal obstruction

Obstructive jaundice
Rarely pancreatitis

Treatment

Palliative treatment for jaundice/cholangitis

Palliative treatment for jaundice

ERCP + stent insertion or percutaneous transhepatic stent insertion

Gastroenterostomy

Definitions

Pancreatic adenocarcinoma is a malignant lesion of the head, body or tail of the pancreas. *Periampullary carcinomas* arise around the ampulla of Vater and include tumours arising from the pancreas, duodenum, distal bile duct and the ampulla itself. *Endocrine pancreatic tumours* cause a variety of syndromes secondary to the secretion of active peptides.

KEY POINTS

- Most pancreatic cancer is not surgically curable.
- New, chronic back pain and vague symptoms may be the only presenting feature.
- The best prognosis is for true periampullary cancers.
- Good palliation of jaundice is possible without surgery.

Epidemiology

Male/female 2 : 1, peak incidence 50–70 years. Incidence of pancreatic carcinoma is increasing in the Western world.

Aetiology

Predisposing factors: smoking, diabetes, chronic pancreatitis.

Pathology

- Site: 55% involve head of pancreas, 25% body, 15% tail, 5% periampullary region.
- Macroscopic: growth is hard and infiltrating.
- Histology: 90% ductal carcinoma, 7% acinar cell carcinoma, 2% cystic carcinoma, 1% connective tissue origins.
- Spread: lymphatics to peritoneum and regional nodes, via bloodstream to liver and lung. Metastases often present at time of diagnosis.

Clinical features

- Head or periampullary: painless, progressive jaundice with a palpable gallbladder (Courvoisier's law: a palpable gallbladder in the presence of jaundice is unlikely to be due to gallstones).
- Occasionally duodenal obstruction causing vomiting.
- Body: back pain, anorexia, weight loss, steatorrhoea.
- Tail: often presents with metastases, malignant ascites or unexplained anaemia.

Investigations

- Ultrasound: may see mass in head of pancreas and distended biliary tree, facilitates needle biopsy.
- CT scan: demonstrates tumour mass, facilitates biopsy, assess involvement of surrounding structures and local lymph node spread.
- ERCP: very accurate in making diagnosis; obtain specimen or shed cells for cytology and stent may be placed to relieve jaundice.
- Barium meal: widening of the duodenal loop with medial filling defect, the reversed '3' sign.

ESSENTIAL MANAGEMENT

Palliation

- Pancreatic adenocarcinoma is usually incurable at time of diagnosis.
- Jaundice can be relieved by placing a stent through the tumour either transhepatically or via ERCP.
- Duodenal obstruction may be relieved by gastrojejunostomy.
- Pain may be helped with a coeliac axis block.

Curative treatment

Rarely surgical (Whipple's) resection of small tumours of the head of the pancreas is curative if lymph nodes are not involved.

Prognosis

- 90% of patients with pancreatic adenocarcinoma are dead within 12 months of diagnosis.
- It is important to obtain histology from tumours around the head of the pancreas as the prognosis from non-pancreatic periampullary cancers is considerably better (50% 5-year survival) following resection.

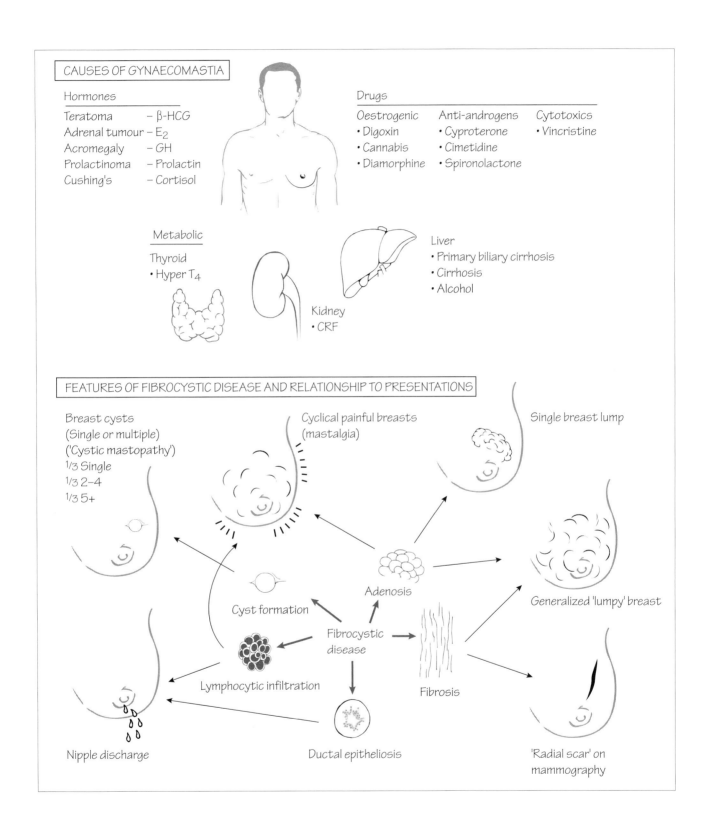

CAUSES OF GYNAECOMASTIA

Hormones

Teratoma	– β-HCG
Adrenal tumour	– E_2
Acromegaly	– GH
Prolactinoma	– Prolactin
Cushing's	– Cortisol

Drugs

Oestrogenic	Anti-androgens	Cytotoxics
• Digoxin	• Cyproterone	• Vincristine
• Cannabis	• Cimetidine	
• Diamorphine	• Spironolactone	

Metabolic

Thyroid
• Hyper T_4

Kidney
• CRF

Liver
• Primary biliary cirrhosis
• Cirrhosis
• Alcohol

FEATURES OF FIBROCYSTIC DISEASE AND RELATIONSHIP TO PRESENTATIONS

Breast cysts
(Single or multiple)
('Cystic mastopathy')
1/3 Single
1/3 2–4
1/3 5+

Cyclical painful breasts
(mastalgia)

Single breast lump

Cyst formation

Adenosis

Generalized 'lumpy' breast

Fibrocystic disease

Lymphocytic infiltration

Fibrosis

Nipple discharge

Ductal epitheliosis

'Radial scar' on mammography

ANDI

Definition

Abnormalities of the Normal Development and Involution of the breast—a broad term covering benign conditions many of which have overlapping features.

Abnormalities of development

Fibroadenoma

• Benign breast lump caused by overgrowth of single breast lobule. Manifests as one or more firm, mobile, painless lumps usually in women under 30 years.
• Investigation: 'triple assessment' (clinical/radiological/cytological) (see p. 121).
• Treatment:
  age <30 either observe or excise if worried;
  age >30 excise to exclude malignancy.

Abnormalities of cycles

Fibrocystic disease

• Usually presents age 25–45 years. May present as breast pain, tenderness, breast lump(s), breast cyst(s), especially during the second half of the menstrual cycle.
• Investigation: 'triple assessment' of all lumps.
• Treatment: patient reassurance, analgesics, γ-linoleic acid, hormone manipulation., cyst aspiration, excision of persistent localized masses after aspiration. Avoid xanthine-containing substances (coffee).

Abnormalities of involution

Breast cyst

• May be single or multiple. Firm, round discrete lump(s).
• Investigation: aspiration ± mammography. Triple assessment for any discrete associated lumps.
• Treatment: reassurance, aspiration (repeated), hormone manipulation.

Other benign conditions

Breast abscess

• Usually infection of the pregnant or lactating breast with *Staphylococcus aureus*. Patient presents with redness, swelling, heat and pain in the breast.

• Treatment is with antibiotics (flucloxacillin) initially but, if an abscess develops, incision and drainage will be required. Lactation/breast feeding does not need to be suppressed while the abscess is being treated.

Mammary duct ectasia

• Dilated subareolar ducts are filled with cellular debris which causes a periductal inflammatory response. Associated with smoking and recurrent non-lactational abscesses. The usual presentation is a green nipple discharge and a subareolar lump.
• Treatment is by subareolar excision of the involved ducts.

Duct papilloma

• Small papillomas arise in the major breast ducts. They cause a bloody or serous nipple discharge.
• Treatment is by excision of the affected duct by microdochectomy.

Fat necrosis

• A fibrous scar in the breast tissue caused by injury, haematoma and necrosis of breast fat with subsequent scarring. History of trauma to the breast in 50% of cases. May be associated with superficial ecchymoses. Histology: periductal cellular infiltrate and fibrosis.
• Investigation: triple assessment.
• Treatment: usually surgical excision to exclude malignancy.

KEY POINTS

• Any breast lump should be evaluated by triple assessment for risk of malignancy whatever the likely diagnosis.
• ANDI disorders are common in younger, premenopausal women and often cause considerable anxiety.
• Gynaecomastia is usually physiological but often needs to be investigated for hormonal causes.

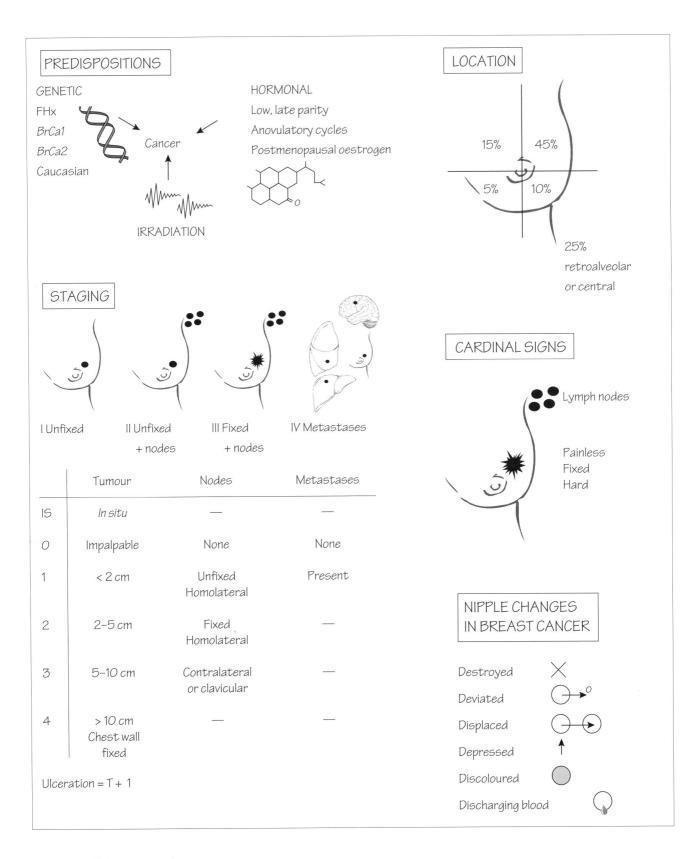

PREDISPOSITIONS

GENETIC
FHx
BrCa1
BrCa2
Caucasian

Cancer

IRRADIATION

HORMONAL
Low, late parity
Anovulatory cycles
Postmenopausal oestrogen

LOCATION

15% 45%

5% 10%

25%
retroalveolar
or central

STAGING

I Unfixed

II Unfixed
+ nodes

III Fixed
+ nodes

IV Metastases

	Tumour	Nodes	Metastases
IS	In situ	—	—
0	Impalpable	None	None
1	< 2 cm	Unfixed Homolateral	Present
2	2–5 cm	Fixed Homolateral	—
3	5–10 cm	Contralateral or clavicular	—
4	> 10 cm Chest wall fixed	—	—

Ulceration = T + 1

CARDINAL SIGNS

Lymph nodes

Painless
Fixed
Hard

NIPPLE CHANGES IN BREAST CANCER

Destroyed

Deviated

Displaced

Depressed

Discoloured

Discharging blood

Definition

Malignant lesion of (predominantly) the female breast.

KEY POINTS

- All breast lumps require triple assessment.
- Early breast cancer can be effectively treated in many cases.
- Early breast cancer treatment is aimed at local control/lymph node treatment and prevention of systemic relapse.
- Treatment of late breast cancer is usually palliative and mostly medical.

Epidemiology

Male/female 1 : 100. Any age (usually >30 years). High incidence in Western world and in white population more than black population.

Aetiology

Predisposing factors:
- strong family history of breast cancer (genetic factors);
- early menarche and late menopause, especially in nulliparous women;
- social class I and II.

Pathology

- Histology: adenocarcinomas arising from the glandular epithelium. Common types are invasive ductal or lobular carcinoma. *Paget's disease* is ductal carcinoma involving the nipple.
- Spread: lymphatics, vascular invasion, direct extension; spreads to lung, liver, bone, brain, adrenal, ovary.
- Staging: TNM classification—important for treatment and prognosis.

Clinical features

- Palpable, hard, irregular, fixed breast lump, usually painless.
- Nipple retraction and skin dimpling.
- Nipple eczema in Paget's disease.
- *Peau d'orange* (cutaneous oedema secondary to lymphatic obstruction).
- Palpable axillary nodes.

Investigations

- Triple assessment: clinical/radiological/cytological.
- Radiological assessment: mammography (ultrasound in young women with dense or large breasts). Features on mammography: irregular, spiculated, radio-opaque mass with microcalcification.
- Cytological assessment: FNAC or core biopsy.
- Breast biopsy: excision biopsy occasionally required for diagnosis.
- Staging investigations for proven carcinoma:
  all: chest X-ray, FBC, serum alkaline phosphatase, γ-glutamyl transpeptidase, serum calcium—(suggest liver or bone metastases);
  if clinically indicated: isotope bone scan, ultrasound scan of liver, brain CT scan.
- Breast tissue for hormone receptor status (ER±), important for treatment and prognosis.

ESSENTIAL MANAGEMENT

Early breast cancer

(No evidence of distant spread at time of diagnosis.)
- Local treatment is usually either:
  lumpectomy + radiotherapy to breast; or
  simple mastectomy.
- Treatment for axillary lymph nodes is usually either:
  axillary dissection (at time of surgery) and removal; or
  radiotherapy to axilla.
- Prevention of systemic spread is usually either:
  hormonal therapy (e.g. tamoxifen); or
  adjuvant chemotherapy (cyclophosphamide, methotrexate, 5-FU) if high risk (positive lymph nodes, bad histological features).
- Prognosis depends on lymph nodes status, tumour size and histological grade: overall 80% 10-year survival rate.

Late breast cancer

(Distant spread at time of diagnosis.)
- Local treatment is directed at controlling local recurrence— lumpectomy/mastectomy/radiotherapy.
- Distant metastases: radiotherapy to relieve pain from bony metastases, chemotherapy (tamoxifen, cytotoxics, aminoglutethamide) to control tumour load.
- Prognosis: poor, only 30–40% respond to treatment with mean survival of 2 years, by which time the non-responders have usually died.

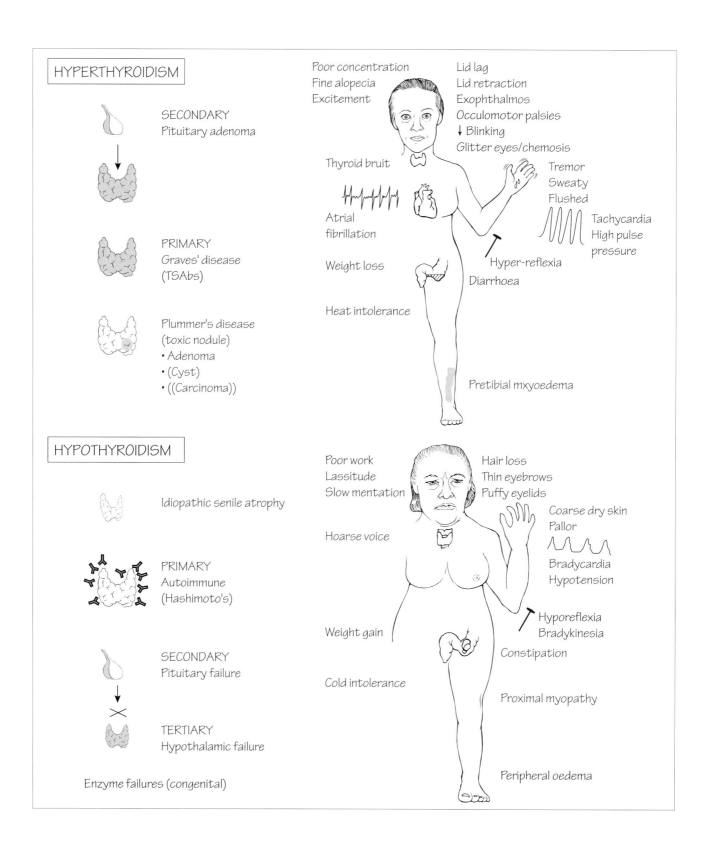

HYPERTHYROIDISM

SECONDARY
Pituitary adenoma

PRIMARY
Graves' disease
(TSAbs)

Plummer's disease
(toxic nodule)
• Adenoma
• (Cyst)
• ((Carcinoma))

Poor concentration
Fine alopecia
Excitement

Lid lag
Lid retraction
Exophthalmos
Occulomotor palsies
↓ Blinking
Glitter eyes/chemosis

Thyroid bruit

Atrial
fibrillation

Weight loss

Heat intolerance

Tremor
Sweaty
Flushed

Tachycardia
High pulse
pressure

Hyper-reflexia

Diarrhoea

Pretibial mxyoedema

HYPOTHYROIDISM

Idiopathic senile atrophy

PRIMARY
Autoimmune
(Hashimoto's)

SECONDARY
Pituitary failure

TERTIARY
Hypothalamic failure

Enzyme failures (congenital)

Poor work
Lassitude
Slow mentation

Hair loss
Thin eyebrows
Puffy eyelids

Hoarse voice

Coarse dry skin
Pallor

Bradycardia
Hypotension

Weight gain

Hyporeflexia
Bradykinesia

Constipation

Cold intolerance

Proximal myopathy

Peripheral oedema

Definition

A goitre is an enlargement of the thyroid gland from any cause.

> **KEY POINTS**
> - Toxic goitres are rarely malignant.
> - All solitary nodules need investigation to exclude carcinoma.
> - Surgery is rarely necessary in autoimmune or inflammatory thyroid disease.

Common causes

- Physiological: gland increases in size as a result of increased demand for thyroid hormone at puberty and during pregnancy.
- Iodine deficiency (endemic): deficiency of iodine results in decreased T_4 levels and increased TSH stimulation leading to a diffuse goitre.
- Primary hyperthyroidism (Graves' disease): goitre and thyrotoxicosis due to circulating immunoglobulin LATS.
- Adenomatous (nodular) goitre: benign hyperplasia of the thyroid gland.
- Thyroiditis: autoimmune (Hashimoto's); subacute (de Quervain's); Riedel's (struma).
- Thyroid malignancies.

Clinical features

Hyperthyroidism

Symptoms
- Heat intolerance and excessive sweating.
- Increased appetite, weight loss, diarrhoea.
- Anxiety, tiredness, palpitations.
- Oligomenorrhoea.

Signs
- Goitre.
- Exophthalmos, lid lag and retraction.
- Warm moist palms, tremor.
- Atrial fibrillation.
- Pretibial myxoedema.

Hypothyroidism

Symptoms
- Cold intolerance, decreased sweating.
- Hoarseness.
- Weight increase, constipation.
- Slow cerebration, tiredness.
- Muscle pains.

Signs
- Pale/yellow skin, dry, thickened skin, thin hair.
- Periorbital puffiness, loss of outer third of eyebrow.
- Dementia, nerve deafness, hyporeflexia.
- Slow pulse, large tongue, peripheral oedema.

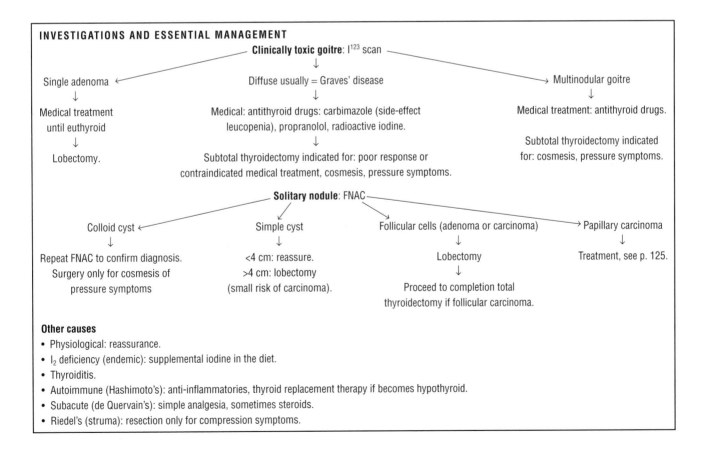

INVESTIGATIONS AND ESSENTIAL MANAGEMENT

Clinically toxic goitre: I^{123} scan

Single adenoma → Diffuse usually = Graves' disease → Multinodular goitre

Medical treatment until euthyroid / Medical: antithyroid drugs: carbimazole (side-effect leucopenia), propranolol, radioactive iodine. / Medical treatment: antithyroid drugs.

Lobectomy. / Subtotal thyroidectomy indicated for: poor response or contraindicated medical treatment, cosmesis, pressure symptoms. / Subtotal thyroidectomy indicated for: cosmesis, pressure symptoms.

Solitary nodule: FNAC

Colloid cyst ← Simple cyst → Follicular cells (adenoma or carcinoma) → Papillary carcinoma

Repeat FNAC to confirm diagnosis. Surgery only for cosmesis of pressure symptoms / <4 cm: reassure. >4 cm: lobectomy (small risk of carcinoma). / Lobectomy → Proceed to completion total thyroidectomy if follicular carcinoma. / Treatment, see p. 125.

Other causes
- Physiological: reassurance.
- I$_2$ deficiency (endemic): supplemental iodine in the diet.
- Thyroiditis.
- Autoimmune (Hashimoto's): anti-inflammatories, thyroid replacement therapy if becomes hypothyroid.
- Subacute (de Quervain's): simple analgesia, sometimes steroids.
- Riedel's (struma): resection only for compression symptoms.

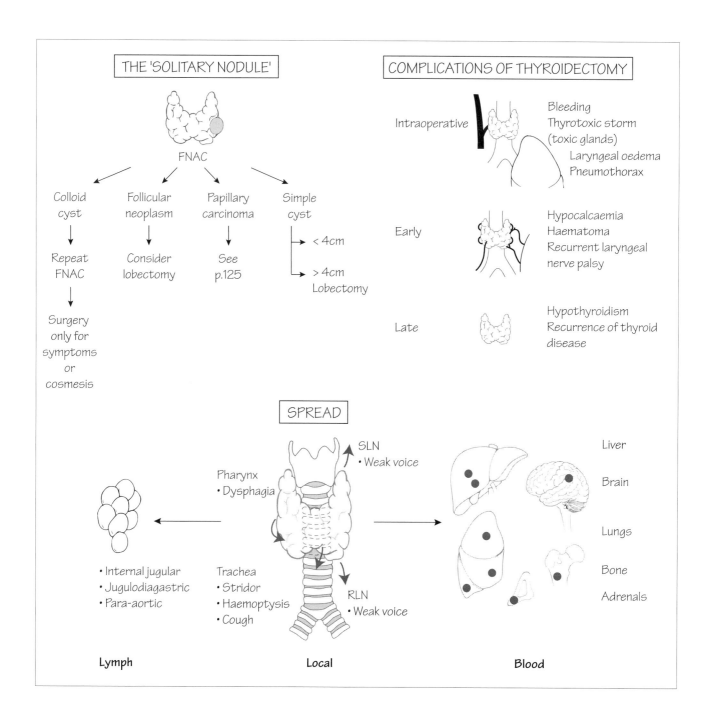

THE 'SOLITARY NODULE'

FNAC

Colloid cyst → Repeat FNAC → Surgery only for symptoms or cosmesis

Follicular neoplasm → Consider lobectomy

Papillary carcinoma → See p.125

Simple cyst → < 4cm / > 4cm Lobectomy

COMPLICATIONS OF THYROIDECTOMY

Intraoperative — Bleeding, Thyrotoxic storm (toxic glands), Laryngeal oedema, Pneumothorax

Early — Hypocalcaemia, Haematoma, Recurrent laryngeal nerve palsy

Late — Hypothyroidism, Recurrence of thyroid disease

SPREAD

SLN • Weak voice
Pharynx • Dysphagia
Trachea • Stridor • Haemoptysis • Cough
RLN • Weak voice

• Internal jugular
• Jugulodiagastric
• Para-aortic

Liver
Brain
Lungs
Bone
Adrenals

Lymph   Local   Blood

Definition

Malignant lesions of the thyroid gland.

KEY POINTS
- Many thyroid tumours are tumours of young adults.
- Isolated thyroid lumps should always be investigated to confirm a cause.
- The prognosis is often good with surgical resection and medical adjuvant treatment.

Epidemiology

Male/female 1 : 2. Peak incidence depends on histology (papillary: young adults; follicular: middle age; anaplastic: elderly; medullary: any age).

Pathology

Histology of thyroid malignancies.

Type	(% of total)	Cell of origin	Differentiation	Spread
Papillary	(60%)	Epithelial	Well	Lymphatic
Follicular	(25%)	Epithelial	Well	Haematogenous
Anaplastic	(10%)	Epithelial	Poor	Direct, lymphatic and haematogenous
Medullary	(5%)	Parafollicular	Moderate	Lymphatic and haematogenous

Aetiology

The following are predisposing factors:
- pre-existing goitre;
- radiation of the neck in childhood.

Clinical features

- Papillary: solitary thyroid nodule.
- Follicular: slow-growing thyroid mass, symptoms from distant metastases.
- Anaplastic: rapidly growing thyroid mass causing tracheal and oesophageal compression.
- Medullary: thyroid lump, may have MEN IIA (medullary thyroid carcinoma, phaeochromocytoma, hyperparathyroidism) or MEN IIB (medullary thyroid carcinoma, phaeochromocytoma, multiple mucosal neuromas, Marfanoid habitus) syndrome.

Investigations

- Ultrasound of the thyroid gland.
- FNAC: may give histological diagnosis.
- Bone scan and radiographs of bones for secondary deposits.
- Calcitonin levels as a marker for medullary carcinoma.

ESSENTIAL MANAGEMENT

Papillary
- Surgery: total thyroidectomy and removal of involved lymph nodes.
- Adjunctive treatment: L-thyroxine postoperatively to suppress TSH production (which stimulates papillary tumour growth).
- Prognosis: excellent.

Follicular
- Surgery: thyroid lobectomy or total thyroidectomy if metastases are present.
- Adjunctive treatment: radioactive iodine (^{131}I) for distant metastases and L-thyroxine for replacement therapy to suppress TSH.
- Prognosis: no metastases—90% 10-year survival; metastases—30% 10-year survival.

Anaplastic
- Surgery: only to relieve pressure symptoms.
- Adjunctive treatment: neither radiotherapy nor chemotherapy is effective.
- Prognosis: dismal—most patients will be dead within 12 months of diagnosis.

Medullary
- Exclude phaeochromocytoma before treating.
- Surgery: total thyroidectomy and excision of regional lymph nodes.
- Prognosis: overall 50% 5-year survival.

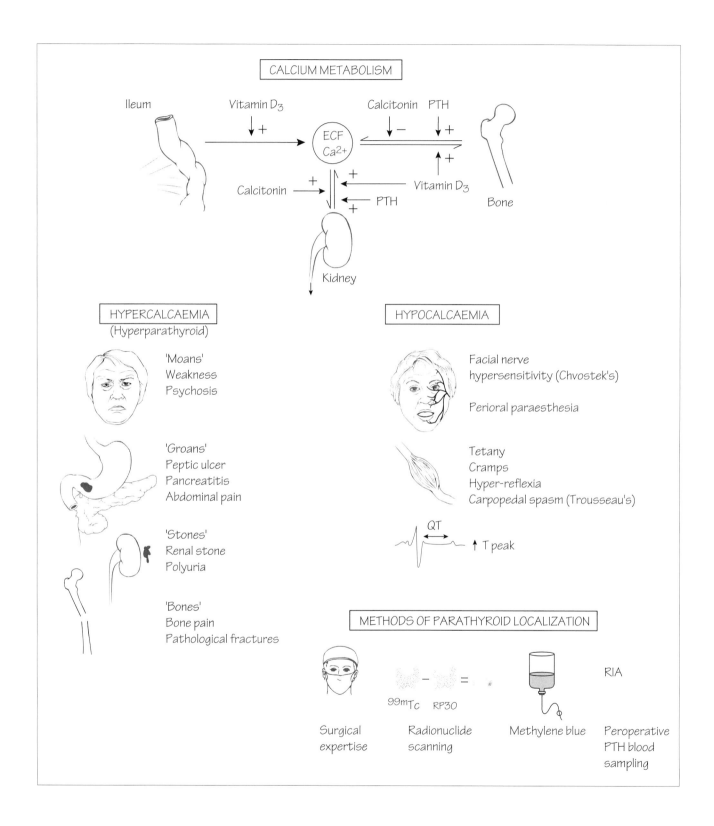

Hyperparathyroidism

Definition

Hyperparathyroidism is a condition characterized by hypercalcaemia caused by excess production of parathyroid hormone.

Causes

• *Primary* hyperparathyroidism is usually due to a parathyroid adenoma (75%) or parathyroid hyperplasia (20%).

• *Secondary* hyperparathyroidism is hyperplasia of the gland in response to hypocalcaemia (e.g. in chronic renal failure).

• In *tertiary* hyperparathyroidism, autonomous secretion of parathormone occurs when the secondary stimulus has been removed (e.g. after renal transplantation).

• *MEN syndromes* and *ectopic* parathormone production (e.g. oat cell carcinoma of the lung).

Pathology

Parathormone mobilizes calcium from bone, enhances renal tubular absorption and, with vitamin D, intestinal absorption of calcium. The net result is *hypercalcaemia*.

Clinical features

• Renal calculi or renal calcification, polyuria.

• Bone pain, bone deformity, osteitis fibrosa cystica, pathological fractures.

• Muscle weakness, anorexia, intestinal atony, psychosis.

• Peptic ulceration and pancreatitis.

Diagnosis

• Serum calcium (specimen taken on three occasions with patient fasting, at rest and without a tourniquet). Normal range 2.2–2.6 mmol/l. Calcium is bound to albumin and the level has to be 'corrected' when albumin levels are abnormal.

• Parathormone level.

• Imaging:

high-resolution ultrasound;

CT and MRI scanning;

dual isotope imaging (^{201}Tl and ^{99m}Tc pertechnate).

• Selective vein catheterization and digital subtraction angiography in patients in whom exploration has been unsuccessful.

ESSENTIAL MANAGEMENT

• Primary and tertiary hyperparathyroidism are treated surgically: excise adenoma if present, remove 3½ of 4 glands for hyperplasia.

• Secondary hyperplasia: vitamin D and/or calcium.

Hypoparathyroidism

Definition

Hypoparathyroidism is a rare condition characterized by hypocalcaemia due to reduced production of parathormone.

Causes

• Post-thyroid or parathyroid surgery.

• Idiopathic (often autoimmune).

• Congenital enzymatic deficiencies.

• Pseudohypoparathyroidism (reduced sensitivity to parathormone).

Pathology

Reduced serum calcium increases neuromuscular excitability.

Clinical features

• Perioral paraesthesia, cramps, tetany.

• *Chvostek's sign*: tapping over facial nerve induces facial muscle contractions.

• *Trousseau's sign*: inflating BP-cuff to above systolic pressure induces typical *main d'accoucheur* carpal spasm.

• Prolonged QT interval on ECG.

Diagnosis

• Calcium and parathormone levels decreased.

ESSENTIAL MANAGEMENT

Calcium and vitamin D.

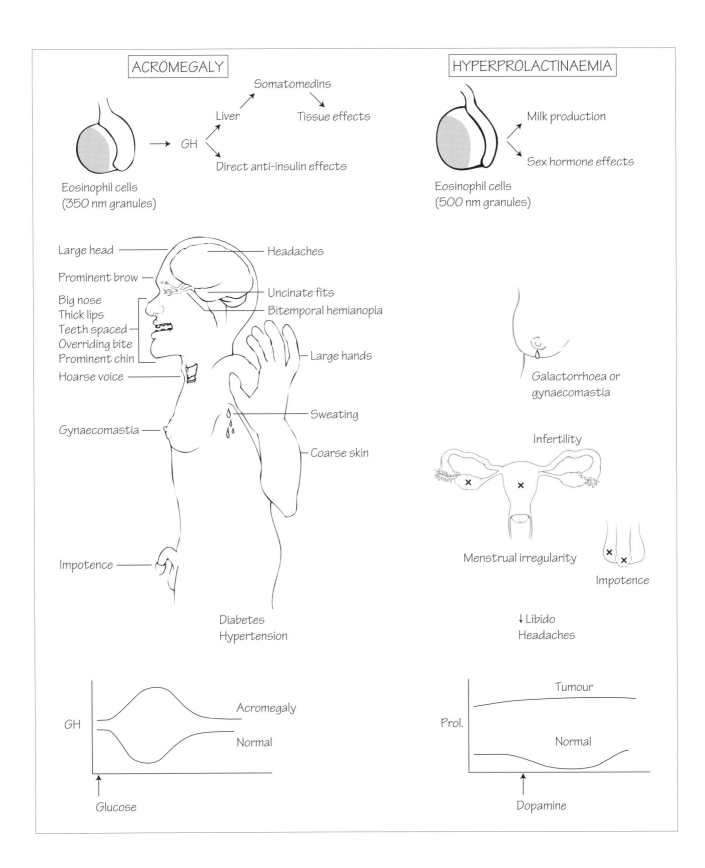

ACROMEGALY

Somatomedins

Liver → Tissue effects

GH

Direct anti-insulin effects

Eosinophil cells
(350 nm granules)

Large head — Headaches
Prominent brow —
Big nose
Thick lips — Uncinate fits
Teeth spaced — Bitemporal hemianopia
Overriding bite
Prominent chin
Hoarse voice — Large hands

Gynaecomastia —
Sweating
Coarse skin

Impotence —

Diabetes
Hypertension

GH
Acromegaly
Normal

Glucose

HYPERPROLACTINAEMIA

Milk production

Sex hormone effects

Eosinophil cells
(500 nm granules)

Galactorrhoea or
gynaecomastia

Infertility

Menstrual irregularity
Impotence

↓ Libido
Headaches

Prol.
Tumour
Normal

Dopamine

Definition

Pituitary disorders are characterized either by a *failure of secretion* of pituitary hormones or by tumours, which cause local pressure effects or specific syndromes due to hormone overproduction.

Common causes

• Failure of anterior pituitary secretion, pan-hypopituitarism (Simmonds' disease):
    pressure from a tumour;
    infection;
    ischaemia;
    postpartum-induced infarction of the anterior pituitary (Sheehan's syndrome).
Failure of antidiuretic hormone production from the posterior pituitary gland leads to diabetes insipidus:
• trauma;
• local haemorrhage;
• ischaemia;
• tumours.

Tumours (% of total)	Cell type
Endocrinologically active (75%)	
Prolactinomas (35%)	Acidophil
GH-secreting tumours (20%)	Acidophil
Mixed PL and GH (10%)	Acidophil
ACTH-secreting tumours (10%)	Basophil
Endocrinologically inactive (25%)	Chromophobe
Craniopharyngioma	Rathke's pouch

Clinical features

• Pan-hypopituitarism: pallor (MSH), hypothyroid (TSH), failure of lactation (PL), chronic adrenal insufficiency (ACTH), ovarian failure and amenorrhoea (FSH, LH).
• Diabetes insipidus (ADH): polyuria (5–20 l/day), polydipsia.
• Tumours: pressure effects: headache, bitemporal hemianopia.
Acromegaly (excess GH): thickened skin, increased skull size, prognathism, enlarged tongue, goitre, osteoporosis, organomegaly, spade-like hands and feet.
Cushing's disease (excess ACTH): malaise, muscle weakness, weight gain, bruising, moon facies, buffalo hump, hirsutism, amenorrhoea, impotence, polyuria, diabetes, emotional instability.

Investigations

• Pan-hypopituitarism: serum assay of pituitary and target gland hormones, dynamic tests of pituitary function.
• Diabetes insipidus: very low urinary specific gravity which does not increase with water deprivation.
• Tumours: visual field measurements, hormone assay, CT or MRI scanning.

ESSENTIAL MANAGEMENT
• Pan-hypopituitarism: replacement therapy—cyclical oestrogen–progesterone, hydrocortisone, thyroxine.
• Diabetes insipidus: vasopressin analogue, desmopressin, administered as nasal spray.
• Tumours: bromocriptine suppresses PL release from prolactinomas, ^{90}Y implant for pituitary ablation, surgery (hypophysectomy via nasal or transcranial route).

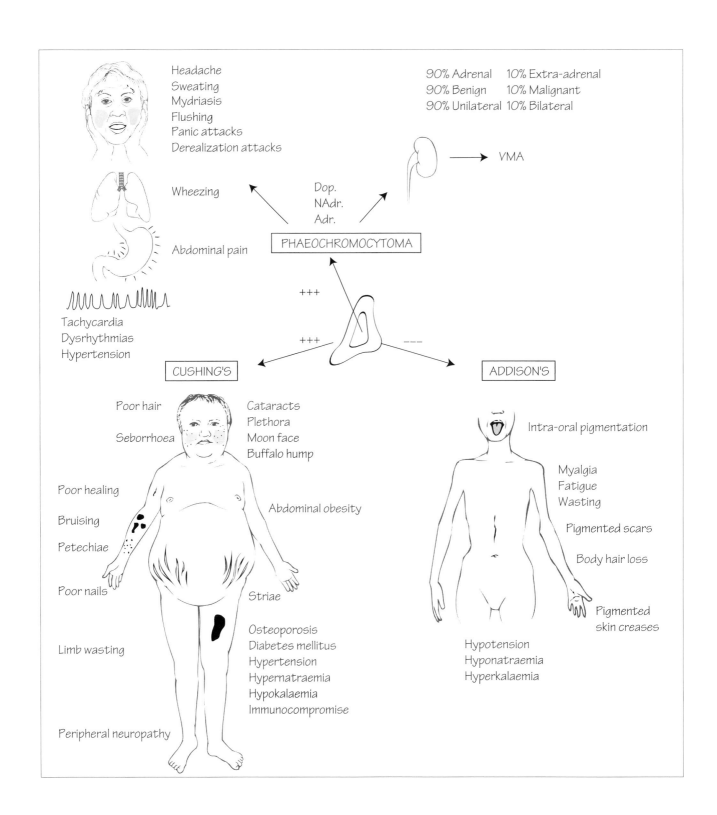

Headache
Sweating
Mydriasis
Flushing
Panic attacks
Derealization attacks

90% Adrenal   10% Extra-adrenal
90% Benign   10% Malignant
90% Unilateral 10% Bilateral

→ VMA

Wheezing

Dop.
NAdr.
Adr.

PHAEOCHROMOCYTOMA

Abdominal pain

+++

+++

Tachycardia
Dysrhythmias
Hypertension

CUSHING'S

ADDISON'S

Poor hair

Cataracts
Plethora
Moon face
Buffalo hump

Seborrhoea

Intra-oral pigmentation

Myalgia
Fatigue
Wasting

Poor healing

Abdominal obesity

Pigmented scars

Bruising

Body hair loss

Petechiae

Poor nails

Striae

Pigmented
skin creases

Limb wasting

Osteoporosis
Diabetes mellitus
Hypertension
Hypernatraemia
Hypokalaemia
Immunocompromise

Hypotension
Hyponatraemia
Hyperkalaemia

Peripheral neuropathy

Definition

Adrenal gland disorders are characterized by clinical syndromes resulting from either a *failure of secretion* or *excessive secretion* of adrenal cortical or medullary hormones.

Cushing's syndrome describes the clinical features irrespective of the cause; *Cushing's disease* refers to a pituitary adenoma with secondary adrenal hyperplasia.

KEY POINTS

- Addison's disease is often insidious in onset and presents with vague symptoms—consider in unexplained lethargy and weakness.
- Phaeochromocytoma can mimic a wide range of acute surgical, medical and psychiatric states.
- Cushing's syndrome is commonly caused by chronic exogenous steroid administration.
- Treatment for most situations aims to normalize body physiology before any definitive/surgical treatment is considered.

Common causes

Failure of secretion

Adrenal insufficiency, Addison's disease: bilateral adrenal haemorrhage in sepsis (Waterhouse–Friderichsen syndrome), autoimmune disease, TB, pituitary insufficiency, metastatic deposits.

Excessive secretion

- Cushing's syndrome: excess corticosteroid due to steroid therapy, ACTH-producing pituitary tumour, adenoma or carcinoma of the adrenal cortex, ectopic ACTH production, e.g. oat-cell carcinoma of lung.
- Conn's syndrome (primary hyperaldosteronism): excess aldosterone due to adenoma or carcinoma of adrenal cortex, bilateral cortical hyperplasia.
- Adrenogenital syndrome: excess androgen: abnormal cortisol synthesis causes excess ACTH production which boosts androgen production, adrenal cortical tumour.
- Phaeochromocytoma: excess catecholamines due to adrenal medullary tumours, 95% are benign.

Clinical features

- Addison's disease: see opposite. Addisonian crisis: an acute collapse which may mimic an abdominal emergency.
- Cushing's syndrome: see opposite.
- Conn's syndrome, primary hyperaldosteronism: muscle weakness, tetany, polyuria, polydipsia, hypertension.
- Adrenogenital syndrome: virilization in female children, pseudohermaphroditism, precocious puberty.
- Phaeochromocytoma: see opposite.

Investigations

Basic principles

- Establish the 'endocrine' diagnosis by serum levels or suppressions/stimulation tests.
- Correct the endocrine abnormalities.
- Localize the cause by investigation and imaging.
- Consider if definitive (surgical) treatment is necessary.

Addison's disease

U+Es ($\downarrow$Na$^+$, $\uparrow$K$^+$), low plasma cortisol, short synacthen test to confirm diagnosis. Long synacthen test to differentiate primary (adrenal) from secondary (pituitary) insufficiency.

Cushing's syndrome

Elevated plasma cortisol (taken at 24.00 hours) and loss of diurnal variation, low-dose dexamethasone suppression test to confirm diagnosis, high-dose test to distinguish adrenal from pituitary disease, serum ACTH to identify secondary cause.

Conn's syndrome

U+Es ($\downarrow$K$^+$, normal or $\uparrow$Na$^+$), raised serum aldosterone and normal renin levels.

Adrenogenital syndrome

Elevated urinary 17 ketosteroids.

Phaeochromocytoma

24-hour urinary VMA, serum dopamine, epinephrine (adrenaline) and norepinephrine (noradrenaline).

Localization imaging

- Helical CT: excellent for adrenal gland, retroperitoneum.
- [^{123}I] MIBG scan: neuroendocrine tumours (phaeochromocytoma).
- Arteriography and venous sampling: occasionally required.

ESSENTIAL MANAGEMENT

- Addison's disease: replacement therapy. Cortisol, fludrocortisone. Increase dose at times of stress/surgery.
- Cushing's syndrome: adrenalectomy for adenoma (rarely carcinoma). Mitotane reduces steroid production in metastases.
- Conn's syndrome: adrenalectomy for unilateral adenoma (rarely carcinoma). Spironolactone or amiloride for bilateral adenomas or hyperplasia. (Only if poor response, bilateral adrenalectomy with replacement therapy.)
- Adrenogenital syndrome: cortisol to suppress ACTH and provide corticosteroids. Surgery to correct abnormalities of external genitalia.
- Phaeochromocytoma: surgery after fluid replacement and careful α and β adrenergic blockade.

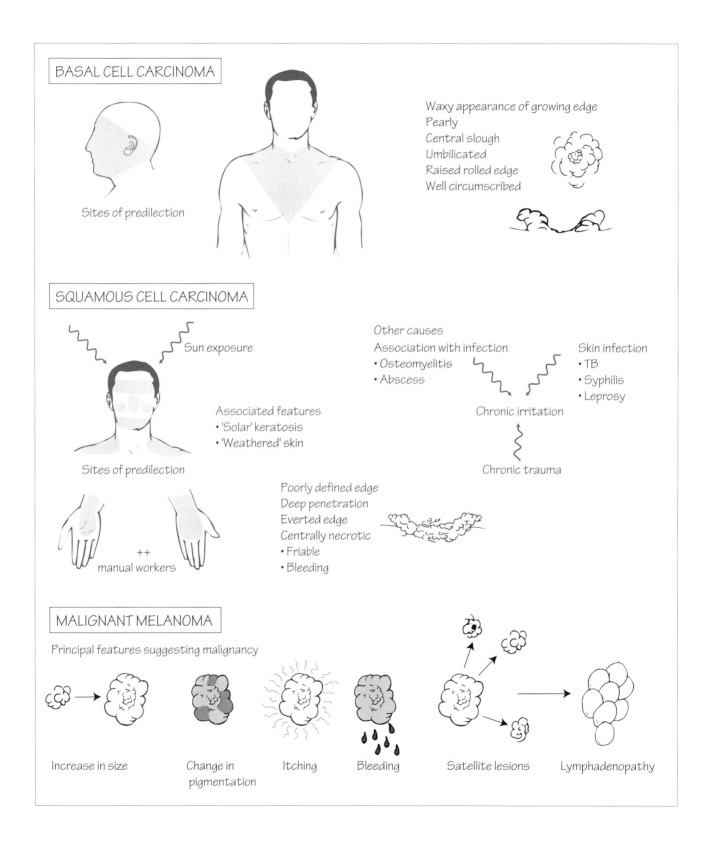

BASAL CELL CARCINOMA

Sites of predilection

Waxy appearance of growing edge
Pearly
Central slough
Umbilicated
Raised rolled edge
Well circumscribed

SQUAMOUS CELL CARCINOMA

Sun exposure

Associated features
• 'Solar' keratosis
• 'Weathered' skin

Sites of predilection

++
manual workers

Other causes
Association with infection
• Osteomyelitis
• Abscess

Skin infection
• TB
• Syphilis
• Leprosy

Chronic irritation

Chronic trauma

Poorly defined edge
Deep penetration
Everted edge
Centrally necrotic
• Friable
• Bleeding

MALIGNANT MELANOMA

Principal features suggesting malignancy

Increase in size | Change in pigmentation | Itching | Bleeding | Satellite lesions | Lymphadenopathy

Definition

Malignant lesions of epidermis of the skin—principally basal cell (BCC) and squamous cell (SCC) carcinomas and malignant melanoma (MM).

> **KEY POINTS**
> • Protection from sun exposure reduces the risk of all forms of skin cancer dramatically.
> • Not all MMs are pigmented.
> • All 'moles' with suspicious features should be *excision* biopsied.
> • The prognosis from early MM is excellent with surgery but late disease is usually fatal.

Epidemiology

Male/female 2 : 1 for BCC and SCC. Elderly males. Equal sex distribution and all adults for MM. All tumours common in areas of high annual sunshine (e.g. Australia, southern USA).

Aetiology

The following are predisposing factors.
• Exposure to sunlight (especially in fair-skinned races).
• Immunosuppression (high incidence after renal transplant).
• Radiation exposure (radiotherapy, among radiologists).
• Chemical carcinogens (hydrocarbons, arsenic, coal tar).
• Inherited disorders (albinism, xeroderma pigmentosum).
• Chronic irritation (Marjolin's ulcer).
• Naevi (50% of MM arise in pre-existing benign pigmented lesions).
• Bowen's disease and erythroplasia of Queryat.

Pathology

BCC
• Arises from basal cells of epidermis.
• Aggressive local spread but do not metastasize.

SCC
• Arises from keratinocytes in the epidermis.
• Spreads by local invasion and metastases.

MM
• Arises from the melanocytes often in pre-existing naevi.
• Superficial spreading and nodular types.
• Radial and vertical growth phases. Lymphatic spread is to regional lymph nodes and haematogenous spread to liver, bone and brain.

Staging

Clarke's levels I–V, Breslow's tumour thickness.

Clinical features

BCC
Recurring, ulcerated, umbilicated skin lesion on forehead or face. Ulcer has a raised, pearl-coloured edge. Untreated, large areas of the face may be eroded (rodent ulcer).

SCC
Lesions (ulcers, fungating lesions with heaped-up edges) on exposed areas of the body.

MM
Pigmented lesions (occasionally not pigmented—amelanotic), 1 cm in diameter on lower limbs, feet, head and neck. Usually present as a change in a pigmented lesion: increasing size or pigmentation/bleeding/pain or itching/ulceration/satellite lesions.

Investigations

• Biopsy (usually excisional) of the lesion unless clinically certain (definitive surgery).
• For MM—helical CT scan for ?involved draining nodes, FNAC for palpable draining nodes, ?peroperative sentinel node biopsy using dye injection mapping.

> **ESSENTIAL MANAGEMENT**
> **BCC**
> • Curettage/cautery/cryotherapy/topical chemotherapy (5-FU). These treatments are suitable for small lesions.
> • Surgical excision/radiotherapy.
>
> **SCC**
> Surgical excision/radiotherapy.
>
> **MM**
> • Surgical excision with 2–3 cm margin.
> • Lymph node dissection if CT, FNAC or sentinel node biopsy +ve for metastases with no systemic disease.
> • Immunotherapy, chemotherapy (systemic and local limb perfusion), radiotherapy disseminated disease (poor response).

Prognosis

• BCC, SCC prognosis is usually excellent, but patients with SCC should be followed for 5 years.
• MM prognosis depends on staging:

Clarke's level	5-year survival (%)	Tumour thickness (mm)	5-year survival (%)
I (epidermis)	100	<0.76	98
II (papillary dermis)	90–100	0.76–1.49	95
III (papillary/reticular dermis)	80–90	1.50–2.49	80
IV (reticular dermis)	60–70	2.50–3.99	75
V (subcutaneous fat)	15–30	4.00–7.99	60
		>8.00	40

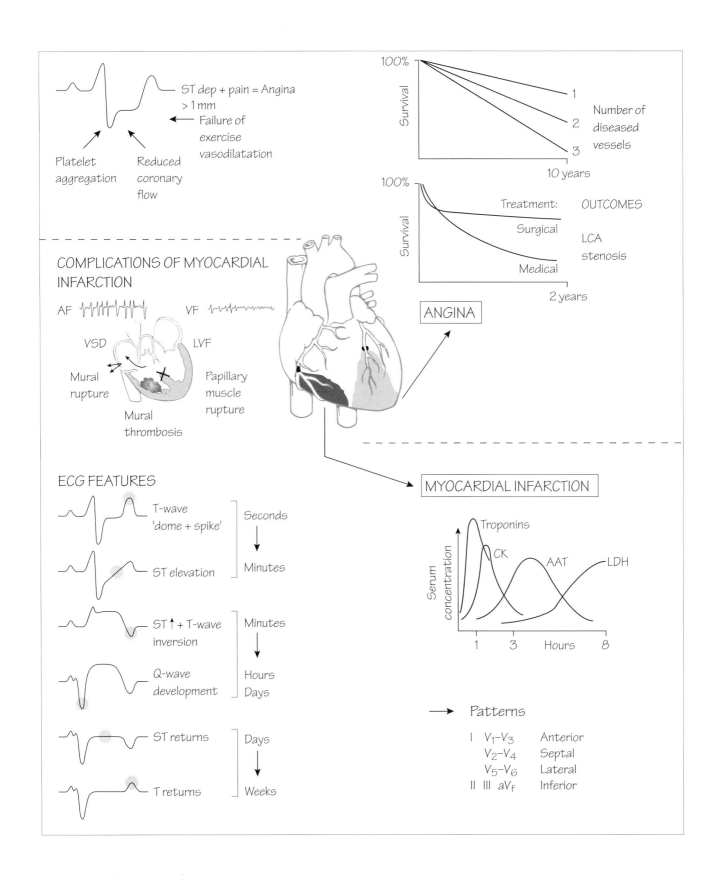

ST dep + pain = Angina
> 1 mm

Failure of exercise vasodilatation

Platelet aggregation

Reduced coronary flow

100%

Survival

1

2

3

Number of diseased vessels

10 years

100%

Survival

Treatment:

Surgical

Medical

OUTCOMES

LCA stenosis

2 years

ANGINA

COMPLICATIONS OF MYOCARDIAL INFARCTION

AF

VF

VSD

LVF

Mural rupture

Papillary muscle rupture

Mural thrombosis

MYOCARDIAL INFARCTION

Serum concentration

Troponins

CK

AAT

LDH

1   3   Hours   8

ECG FEATURES

T-wave 'dome + spike'   Seconds

ST elevation   Minutes

ST↑ + T-wave inversion   Minutes

Q-wave development   Hours Days

ST returns   Days

T returns   Weeks

Patterns

I	V_1–V_3	Anterior
	V_2–V_4	Septal
	V_5–V_6	Lateral
II III aV$_f$		Inferior

Definition

Ischaemic heart disease is a common disorder caused by acute or chronic interruption of the blood supply to the myocardium, usually due to atherosclerosis of the coronary arteries, i.e. *coronary artery disease*.

> **KEY POINTS**
> • Angina alone is rarely managed surgically (CABG).
> • Urgent treatment with thrombolysis, antiplatelet agents and cardioprotection reduces the risk of death from MI significantly.
> • Serum troponins are highly sensitive and very specific for myocardial injury.

Epidemiology

Male > female before 65 years. Increasing risk with increasing age up to 80 years. Commonest cause of death in the Western world.

Aetiology

- Atherosclerosis and thrombosis.
- Thromboemboli (especially plaque rupture).
- Arteritis (e.g. periarteritis nodosa).
- Coronary artery spasm.
- Extension of aortic dissection/syphilitic aortitis.

Risk factors

- Family history.
- Cigarette smoking.
- Hypertension.
- Hyperlipidaemia.
- 'Type A' personality.
- Obesity.

Pathology

- Reduction in coronary blood flow is critical when lumen is decreased by 90%.
- Angina pectoris results when the supply of O_2 to the heart muscle is unable to meet the increased demands for O_2, e.g. during exercise, cold, after a meal.
- Thrombotic occlusion of the narrowed lumen precipitates acute ischaemia.
- The heart muscle in the territory of the occluded vessel dies, i.e. MI. May be subendocardial or transmural.

Clinical features

Angina pectoris

- Central chest pain on exertion, especially in cold weather, lasts 1–15 min.
- Radiates to neck, jaw, arms.
- Relieved by GTN.
- Usually no signs.

Myocardial infarction

- Severe central chest pain for >30 min duration.
- Radiates to neck, jaw, arms.
- Not relieved by GTN.
- Signs of cardiogenic shock.
- Arrhythmias.

Investigations

Angina pectoris

- FBC: anaemia.
- Thyroid function tests.
- Chest X-ray: heart size.
- ECG ST segment changes.
- Exercise ECG.
- Coronary angiography.

Myocardial infarction

- ECG: Q waves, ST segment and T-wave changes.
- Cardiac enzymes: troponins, LDH, CPK (MB).
- Chest X-ray: dissection.
- FBC: associated anaemia.
- U+E: kyperkalaemia.

> **ESSENTIAL MANAGEMENT**
>
> **Angina pectoris**
> - Lose weight.
> - Avoid precipitating factors (e.g. cold).
> - GTN (sublingual).
> - Calcium channel blockers.
> - β-blockers, nitrates, aspirin.
> - Treatment of hypertension and hyperlipidaemias.
> - Coronary angioplasty or CABG.
>
> **Myocardial infarction**
> - Bed rest, O_2, analgesia.
> - Thrombolysis.
> - Aspirin.
> - Treatment of heart failure.
> - Treatment of arrhythmias.
>
> **Indications for CABG**
> - Left main stem disease.
> - Triple vessel disease.
> - Two-vessel disease involving LAD.
> - Chronic ischaemia + LV dysfunction.

Complications of MI

- Arrhythmias.
- Cardiogenic shock.
- Myocardial rupture.
- Papillary muscle rupture causing mitral incompetence.
- Ventricular aneurysm.
- Pericarditis.
- Mural thrombosis and peripheral embolism.

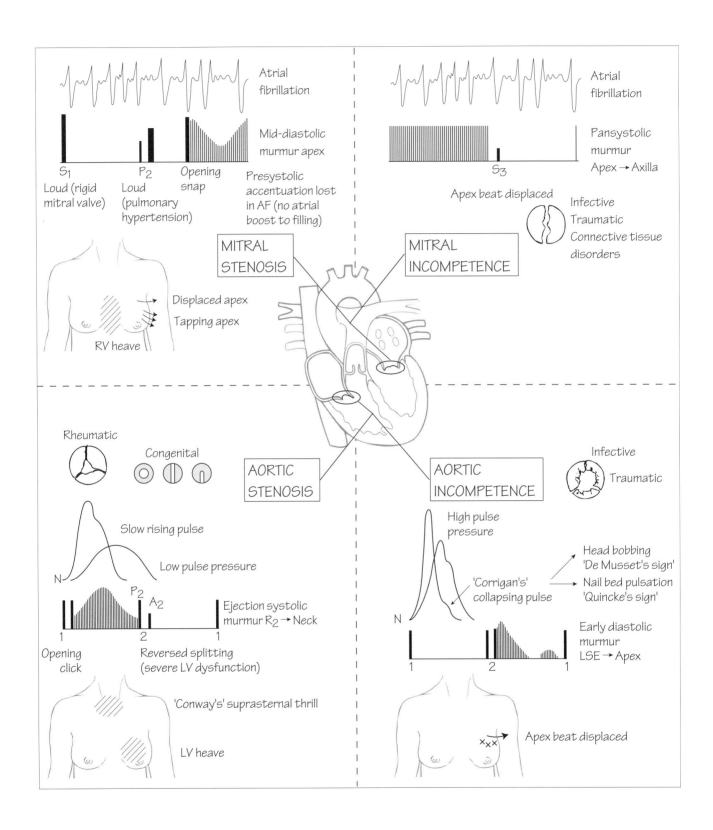

Atrial fibrillation

S_1
Loud (rigid mitral valve)

P_2
Loud (pulmonary hypertension)

Opening snap

Mid-diastolic murmur apex

Presystolic accentuation lost in AF (no atrial boost to filling)

MITRAL STENOSIS

Displaced apex
Tapping apex
RV heave

Atrial fibrillation

S_3

Pansystolic murmur
Apex → Axilla

Apex beat displaced

Infective
Traumatic
Connective tissue disorders

MITRAL INCOMPETENCE

Rheumatic

Congenital

Slow rising pulse

Low pulse pressure

P_2 A_2

Ejection systolic murmur R_2 → Neck

1   2   1

Opening click

Reversed splitting (severe LV dysfunction)

AORTIC STENOSIS

'Conway's' suprasternal thrill

LV heave

Infective

Traumatic

High pulse pressure

'Corrigan's' collapsing pulse

Head bobbing 'De Musset's sign'

Nail bed pulsation 'Quincke's sign'

Early diastolic murmur LSE → Apex

1   2   1

AORTIC INCOMPETENCE

Apex beat displaced

Definition

Valvular heart disease is defined as a group of conditions characterized by damage to one or more of the heart valves, resulting in deranged blood flow through the heart chambers.

Epidemiology

Rheumatic fever is still a major problem in developing countries, while congenital heart disease occurs in 8–10 cases per 1000 live births worldwide.

Aetiology

- Congenital valve abnormalities.
- Rheumatic fever.
- Infective endocarditis.
- Degenerative valve disease.

Pathology

- Rheumatic fever—*immune-mediated acute inflammation* affecting the heart valves due to a cross-reaction between antigens of group A α-haemolytic *Streptococcus* and cardiac proteins.
- Disease may make the valve orifice smaller (*stenosis*) or unable to close properly (*incompetence* or *regurgitation*) or both.
- Stenosis causes a *pressure load* while regurgitation causes a *volume load* on the heart chamber immediately proximal to it with upstream and downstream effects.

Clinical features

Aortic stenosis

- Angina pectoris.
- Syncope.
- Left heart failure.
- Slow upstroke arterial pulse.
- Precordial systolic thrill (second right ICS).
- Harsh midsystolic ejection murmur (second right ICS).

Aortic regurgitation

- Congestive cardiac failure.
- Increased pulse pressure.
- Water-hammer pulse.
- Decrescendo diastolic murmur (lower left sternal edge).

Mitral stenosis

- Pulmonary hypertension.
- Paroxysmal nocturnal dyspnoea.
- Atrial fibrillation.
- Loud first heart sound and opening snap.
- Low-pitched diastolic murmur with presystolic accentuation at the apex.

Mitral regurgitation

- Chronic fatigue.
- Pulmonary oedema.
- Apex laterally displaced, hyperdynamic praecordium.
- Apical pansystolic murmur radiating to axilla.

Tricuspid stenosis

- Fatigue.
- Peripheral oedema.
- Liver enlargement/ascites.
- Prominent JVP with large a waves.
- Lung fields are clear.
- Rumbling diastolic murmur (lower left sternal border).

Tricuspid regurgitation

- Chronic fatigue.
- Hepatomegaly/ascites.
- Right ventricular heave.
- Prominent JVP with large v waves.
- Pansystolic murmur (subxiphoid area).

Investigations

- ECG.
- Chest X-ray.
- Echocardiography and colour Doppler techniques.
- Cardiac catheterization with measurement of transvalvular gradients.

ESSENTIAL MANAGEMENT

Medical

Treat cardiac failure, diuretics, restrict salt intake, reduce exercise, digitalis for rapid atrial fibrillation and anticoagulation for peripheral embolization.

Surgical

Repair (possible in mitral and tricuspid valve only) or replace diseased valve (requires cardiopulmonary bypass). *Prosthetic* (lifelong anticoagulation), *bioprosthetic* (animal tissue on prosthetic frame, 3 months' anticoagulation) and *biological* (cadaveric homografts, no anticoagulation) valves available.

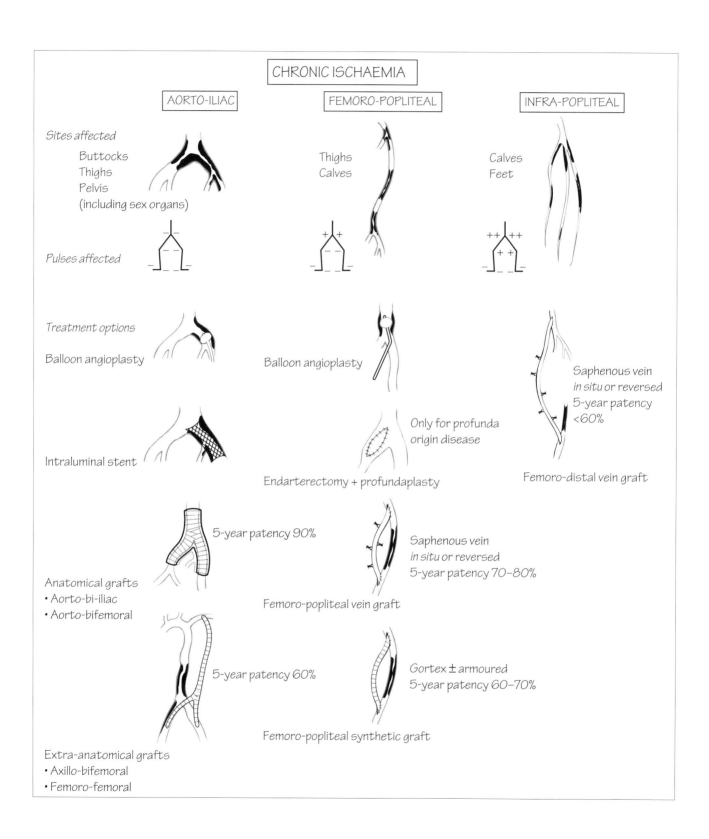

Definition

Peripheral occlusive vascular disease (POVD) is a common disorder caused by acute or chronic interruption of the blood supply to the limbs, usually due to atherosclerosis.

> **KEY POINTS**
> - All patients with POVD require screening for associated coronary or carotid disease.
> - The majority of POVD responds to conservative treatment.
> - Surgery is confined to limb-threatening (critical) ischaemia or truly disabling, refractory claudication.

Epidemiology

Male > female before 65 years. Increased risk with increased age.

Aetiology

- Atherosclerosis and thrombosis.
- Embolism.
- Vascular trauma.
- Vasculitis (e.g. Buerger's disease).

Risk factors

- Cigarette smoking.
- Hypertension.
- Hyperlipidaemia.
- Diabetes mellitus.
- Family history.

Pathology

Reduction in blood flow to the peripheral tissues results in ischaemia which may be acute or chronic. Critical ischaemia is present when the reduction of blood flow is such that tissue viability cannot be sustained (defined by tissue loss, rest pain for 2 weeks, ankle pressure <50 mmHg).

Clinical features

Chronic ischaemia (see p. 50)

- Intermittent claudication in calf (femoral), thigh (iliac) or buttock (aortoiliac).
- Cold peripheries.
- Prolonged capillary refill time.
- Rest pain, especially at night.
- Venous guttering.
- Absent pulses.
- Arterial ulcers, especially over pressure points (heels, toes).
- Knee contractures.

Acute ischaemia (see p. 54)

- Pain.
- Pallor.
- Pulselessness.
- Paraesthesia.
- Paralysis.
- 'Perishing' cold.
- 'Pistol shot' onset.
- Mottling.
- Muscle rigidity.

Investigations

Chronic ischaemia

- ABI (normal >1.0) at rest and postexercise on treadmill.
- FBC (exclude polycythaemia).
- Doppler wave-form analysis.
- Digital plethysmography (in diabetes).
- Perfemoral angiography.

Acute ischaemia

- ECG, cardiac enzymes.
- Angiography (?), may be performed peroperatively.
- Find source of embolism. Holter monitoring. Echocardiograph. Ultrasound aorta for AAA.

ESSENTIAL MANAGEMENT

Non-disabling claudication

- Stop smoking.
- Exercise programme.
- Avoid β-blockers.
- Aspirin 75 mg/day; clopidogril 75 mg/day.
- Pentoxifylline (?).
- Lipid-lowering drug if hyperlipidaemia present.

Disabling claudication/critical ischaemia

- Balloon angioplasty ± intravascular stent.
- Bypass surgery.
- Amputation.
- i.v. treatment: iloprost.

Acute ischaemia

- Heparin anticoagulation.
- Surgical embolectomy.
- Thrombolytic therapy (t-PA, streptokinase, urokinase).

Prognosis

Non-disabling claudication

>65% respond to conservative management. The rest require more aggressive treatment.

Disabling claudication/critical ischaemia

- Angioplasty and bypass surgery overall give good results.
- The more distal the anastomosis the poorer the result.

Acute ischaemia

- Limb salvage 85%.
- Mortality 10–15%.

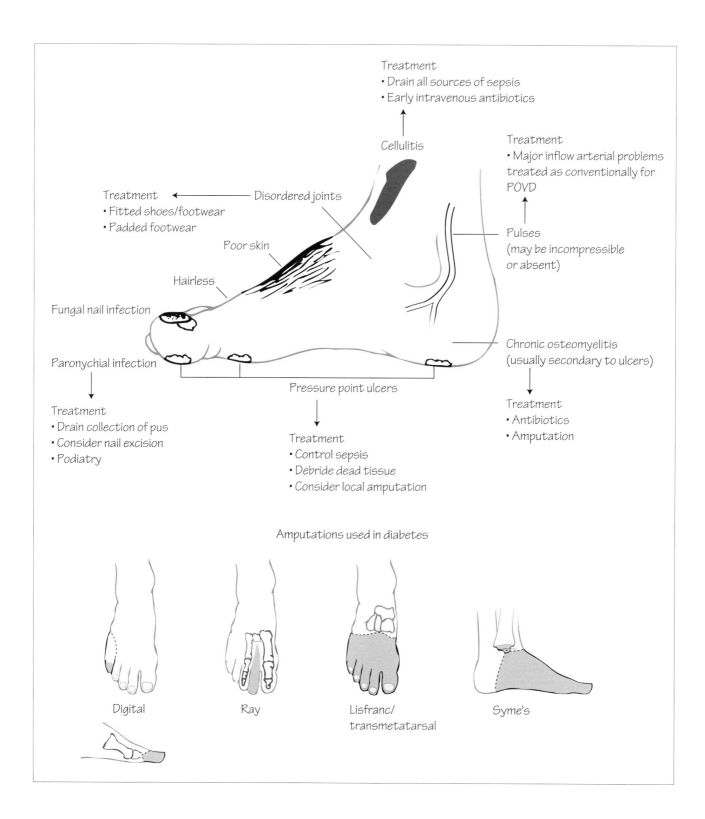

Treatment
• Drain all sources of sepsis
• Early intravenous antibiotics

Cellulitis

Treatment
• Major inflow arterial problems treated as conventionally for POVD

Treatment ←── Disordered joints
• Fitted shoes/footwear
• Padded footwear

Pulses
(may be incompressible or absent)

Poor skin

Hairless

Fungal nail infection

Paronychial infection

Chronic osteomyelitis
(usually secondary to ulcers)

Pressure point ulcers

Treatment
• Drain collection of pus
• Consider nail excision
• Podiatry

Treatment
• Antibiotics
• Amputation

Treatment
• Control sepsis
• Debride dead tissue
• Consider local amputation

Amputations used in diabetes

Digital   Ray   Lisfranc/   Syme's
                              transmetatarsal

Definition

The term *diabetic foot* refers to a spectrum of foot disorders ranging from ulceration to gangrene occurring in diabetic people as a result of peripheral neuropathy or ischaemia, or both.

KEY POINTS
- Prevention is everything in diabetic feet.
- All infections should be treated aggressively to reduce the risk of tissue loss.
- Treat major vessel POVD as normal—improve 'inflow' to the foot.

Pathophysiology

Three distinct processes lead to the problem of the diabetic foot.
- *Ischaemia* caused by macro- and microangiopathy.
- *Neuropathy*: sensory, motor and autonomic.
- *Sepsis*: the glucose-saturated tissue promotes bacterial growth.

Clinical features

Neuropathic features

- Sensory disturbances.
- Trophic skin changes.
- Plantar ulceration.
- Degenerative arthropathy (Charcot's joints).
- Pulses often present.
- Sepsis (bacterial/fungal).

Ischaemic features

- Rest pain.
- Painful ulcers over pressure areas.
- History of intermittent claudication.
- Absent pulses.
- Sepsis (bacterial/fungal).

Investigations

- Non-invasive vascular tests: ABI, segmental pressure, digital pressure. ABI may be falsely elevated due to medial sclerosis.
- X-ray of foot may show osteomyelitis.
- Arteriography.

ESSENTIAL MANAGEMENT

Should be undertaken jointly by surgeon and physician as diabetic foot may precipitate diabetic ketoacidosis.

Prevention

Do
- Carefully wash and dry feet daily.
- Inspect feet daily.
- Take meticulous care of toenails.
- Use antifungal powder.

Do not
- Walk barefoot.
- Wear ill-fitting shoes.
- Use a hot water bottle.
- Ignore any foot injury.

Neuropathic disease
- Control infection with antibiotics effective against both aerobes and anaerobes.
- Wide local excision and drainage of necrotic tissue.
- These measures usually result in healing.

Ischaemic disease
- Formal assessment of the vascular tree by angiography and reconstitution of the blood supply to the foot (either by angioplasty or bypass surgery) must be achieved before the local measures will work.
- After restoration of blood supply treat as for neuropathic disease.

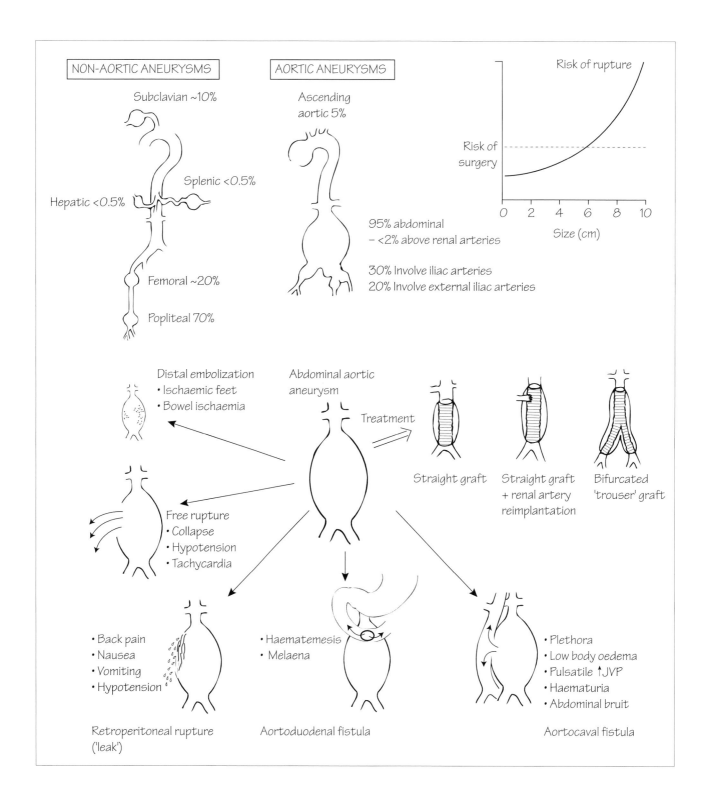

Definition

An *aneurysm* is a permanent localized dilatation of an artery to the extent that the affected artery is 1.5 times its normal diameter. A *pseudo* or *false aneurysm* is an expanding pulsating haematoma in continuity with a vessel lumen. It does not have an epithelial lining.

> **KEY POINTS**
> - All patients with other vascular disease should be examined for AAA.
> - Regular monitoring of size helps determine timing for elective surgery.
> - Mortality for elective surgery is reduced by careful patient evaluation for hidden coronary or pulmonary disease.

Sites

Abdominal aorta, iliac, femoral and popliteal arteries. Cerebral and thoracic aneurysms are less common.

Aetiology

- Atherosclerosis.
- Familial (abnormal collagenase or elastase activity).
- Congenital (cerebral (berry) aneurysm).
- Bacterial aortitis (mycotic aneurysm).
- Syphilitic aortitis (thoracic aneurysm).

Risk factors

- Cigarette smoking.
- Hypertension.
- Hyperlipidaemia.

Pathology

- Aneurysms increase in size in line with the law of Laplace ($T = RP$), T = tension on the arterial wall, R = radius of artery, P = blood pressure. Increasing tension leads to rupture.
- Thrombus from within an aneurysm may be a source of peripheral emboli.
- Popliteal aneurysms may undergo complete thrombosis leading to acute leg ischaemia.
- Aneurysms may be fusiform (AAA, popliteal) or saccular (thoracic, cerebral).

Clinical features of AAA

Asymptomatic

The vast majority have no symptoms and are found incidentally. This has led to the description of an AAA as 'a U-boat in the belly'.

Symptomatic

- Back pain from pressure on the vertebral column.
- Rapid expansion causes flank or back pain.
- Rupture causes collapse, back pain and an ill-defined mass.
- Erosion into IVC causes CCF, loud abdominal bruit, lower limb ischaemia and gross oedema.

Investigations

Detection of AAA

- Physical examination: not accurate.
- Plain abdominal X-ray: aortic calcification.
- Ultrasonography: best way of detecting and measuring aneurysm size.
- CT scan: provides good information regarding relationship between AAA and renal arteries.
- Angiography: not routine for AAA.

Determination of fitness for surgery

- History and examination.
- ECG ± stress testing.
- Radionuclide cardiac scanning (MUGA or stress thallium scan).
- Pulmonary function tests.
- U+E and creatinine for renal assessment.

> **ESSENTIAL MANAGEMENT**
> - Surgical repair is the treatment of choice for AAA.
> - AAA of ≥5.5 cm should be repaired electively as they have a high rate of rupture (perioperative mortality for elective AAA repair is 5%).
> - Surgical repair with *inlay of a synthetic graft* is the standard method of repair.
> - Endovascular repair with graft/stent devices is indicated in selected patients.
> - *Ruptured AAA* require immediate surgical repair (perioperative mortality 50%, but 70% of patients die before they get to hospital so that overall mortality is 85%).

Prognosis

Most patients do well after surviving AAA repair and have an excellent quality of life.

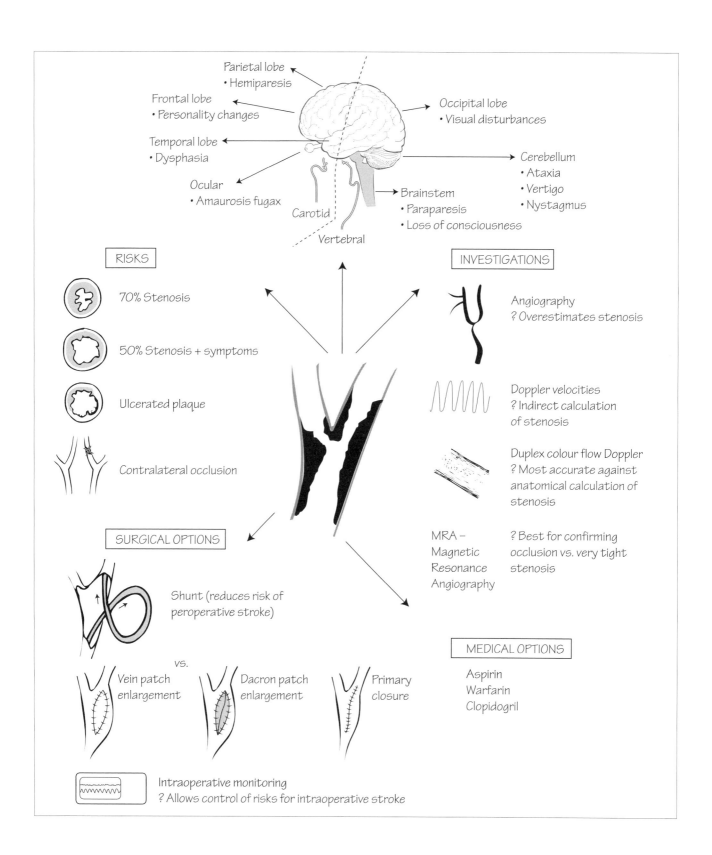

Parietal lobe
• Hemiparesis

Frontal lobe
• Personality changes

Temporal lobe
• Dysphasia

Ocular
• Amaurosis fugax

Carotid

Vertebral

Occipital lobe
• Visual disturbances

Cerebellum
• Ataxia
• Vertigo
• Nystagmus

Brainstem
• Paraparesis
• Loss of consciousness

RISKS

70% Stenosis

50% Stenosis + symptoms

Ulcerated plaque

Contralateral occlusion

INVESTIGATIONS

Angiography
? Overestimates stenosis

Doppler velocities
? Indirect calculation
of stenosis

Duplex colour flow Doppler
? Most accurate against
anatomical calculation of
stenosis

MRA –
Magnetic
Resonance
Angiography

? Best for confirming
occlusion vs. very tight
stenosis

SURGICAL OPTIONS

Shunt (reduces risk of
peroperative stroke)

vs.

Vein patch
enlargement

Dacron patch
enlargement

Primary
closure

MEDICAL OPTIONS

Aspirin
Warfarin
Clopidogril

Intraoperative monitoring
? Allows control of risks for intraoperative stroke

Definition

Extracranial arterial disease is a common disorder characterized by atherosclerosis of the carotid or vertebral arteries resulting in cerebral-ocular (*stroke, TIA, amaurosis fugax*) or cerebellar (vertigo, ataxia, drop attacks) ischaemic symptoms.

> **KEY POINTS**
> * All patients with transient neurological symptoms should undergo screening for carotid disease—clinical examination is not accurate.
> * Targeted carotid endarterectomy offers optimal risk benefit in stroke prevention.

Epidemiology

Male > female before 65 years. Increasing risk with increasing age.

Aetiology

* Atherosclerosis and thrombosis.
* Thromboemboli.
* Fibromuscular dysplasia.

Risk factors

* Cigarette smoking.
* Hypertension.
* Hyperlipidaemia.

Pathophysiology

* The commonest extracranial lesion is an atherosclerotic plaque at the carotid bifurcation. Platelet aggregation and subsequent *platelet embolization* cause ocular or cerebral symptoms.
* Symptoms due to *flow reduction* are rare in the carotid territory, but vertebrobasilar symptoms are usually flow related. Reversed flow in the vertebral artery in the presence of ipsilateral subclavian occlusion leads to cerebral symptoms as the arm 'steals' blood from the cerebellum—subclavian steal syndrome.

Clinical features

* Cerebral symptoms (contralateral):
  motor (weakness, clumsiness or paralysis of a limb);
  sensory (numbness, paraesthesia);
  speech related (receptive or expressive dysphasia).
* Ocular symptoms (ipsilateral): amaurosis fugax (transient loss of vision described as a veil coming down over the visual field).
* Cerebral (or ocular) symptoms may be transitory (a *transient ischaemic attack* is a focal neurological or ocular deficit lasting not more than 24 hours) or permanent (a *stroke*).
* Vertebrobasilar symptoms: vertigo, ataxia, dizziness, syncope, bilateral paraesthesia, visual hallucinations.
* A *bruit* may be heard over a carotid artery, but it is an unreliable indicator of pathology.

Investigations

* Duplex scanning: B-mode scan and Doppler ultrasonic velocitometry: method of choice for assessing degree of carotid stenosis.
* Carotid angiography: no longer essential prior to surgery.
* CT or MRI brain scan: demonstrate the presence of a cerebral infarct.

ESSENTIAL MANAGEMENT

Medical
* Aspirin (75 mg/day) inhibits platelet aggregation for the life of the platelet.
* Clopidogril has a similar action to aspirin.
* Anticoagulation is indicated in patients with cardiac embolic disease.

Surgical
* Carotid endarterectomy (+ aspirin).

Indications for carotid endarterectomy
* Carotid distribution TIA or stroke with good recovery after 1-month delay:
  >70% ipsilateral stenosis;
  >50% ipsilateral stenosis with ulceration.
* Asymptomatic carotid stenosis >80% (controversial).
* Carotid endarterectomy has about 5% morbidity and mortality.
* Carotid angioplasty ± stenting—controversial.

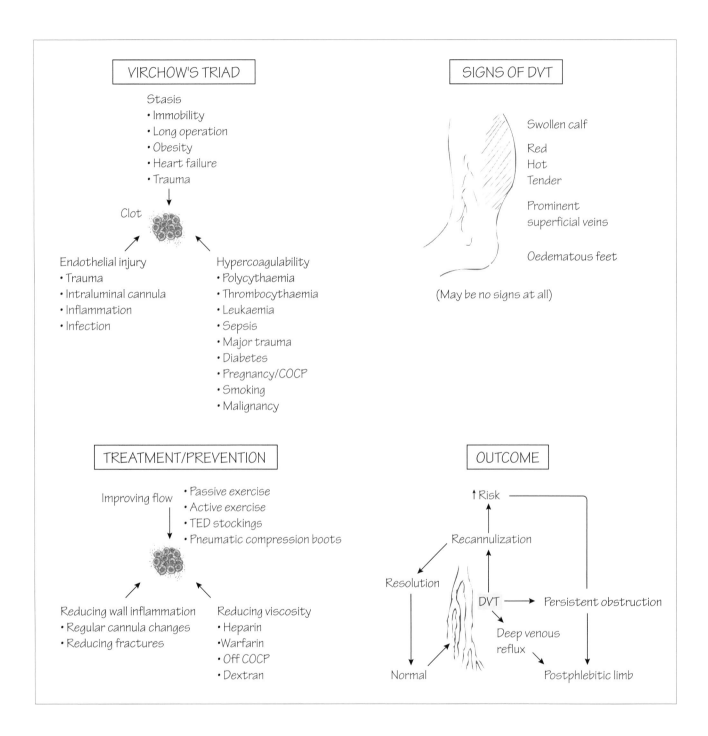

Definitions

A *deep venous thrombosis* (DVT) is a condition in which the blood in the deep veins of the legs or pelvis clots. Embolization of the thrombus results in a *pulmonary embolus* (PE) while local venous damage may lead to chronic venous hypertension and the *postphlebitic limb* (PPL).

KEY POINTS

- All patients in hospital should be considered for mechanical and pharmacological DVT prophylaxis.
- Have a low threshold of investigation for DVT in bed-bound patients.
- Recurrent DVT may lead to chronic disabling postphlebitic limb.
- DVT may be the first manifestation of an occult malignancy.

Epidemiology

DVT is extremely common among medical and surgical patients, affecting 10–30% of all general surgical patients over 40 years who undergo a major operation. PE is a common cause of sudden death in hospital patients (0.5–3.0% of patients die from PE).

Aetiology

Risk factors

- Increasing age >40 years.
- Immobilization.
- Obesity.
- Malignancy.
- Sepsis.
- Thrombophilia (e.g. antithrombin III/protein C/protein S deficiency, Factor V leiden, anticardiolipin Ab).
- Inflammatory bowel disease.
- Trauma.
- Heart disease.
- Pregnancy/oestrogens.

Virchow's triad

- Stasis.
- Endothelial injury.
- Hypercoagulability.

Pathology

- Aggregation of platelets in valve pockets (area of maximum stasis or injury).
- Activation of clotting cascade producing fibrin.
- Fibrin production overwhelms the natural anticoagulant/fibrinolytic system.
- Natural history.
- Complete resolution vs. PE vs. PPL.

Clinical features

DVT

- Asymptomatic.
- Calf tenderness, ankle oedema, mild pyrexia,
- Phlegmasia alba/caerulea dolens.

PE

- Substernal chest pain.
- Dyspnoea.
- Circulatory arrest.
- Pleuritic chest pain.
- Haemoptysis.

PPL

- History of DVT.
- Aching limb.
- Leg swelling.
- Venous eczema.
- Venous ulceration.
- Inverted bottle-shaped leg.

Investigations

DVT

- D-dimers.
- Duplex imaging—suprapopliteal thrombosis.
- Ascending venography.

PE

- ECG: S1, Q3, T3.
- Chest X-ray: linear collapse.
- Blood gases: hypoxia, hypocapnia.
- Ventilation/perfusion lung scan.
- Pulmonary angiography.

PPL

- Ascending ± descending venography.
- Duplex scanning.
- Plethysmography.
- Ambulatory venous pressure.

ESSENTIAL MANAGEMENT

Prophylaxis against DVT

Indications

Presence of risk factors (see above).

Methods

- Mechanical compression (TED) stockings.
- Pharmacological subcutaneous heparin 5000 iu s.c. b.d. (warfarin 1 mg/day, dextran 70 i.v., 500 ml/day).

Definitive treatment

DVT

- Anticoagulation for 6–8 weeks:
  i.v. heparin (check efficacy with APTT);
  warfarin (check efficacy with PT).
- (• Thrombolysis.)
- (• Thrombectomy.)

PE

- Anticoagulation for 3–6 months.
- Thrombolysis.
- Pulmonary embolectomy.
- IVC filters for recurrent PE despite treatment, anticoagulation treatment contraindicated, 'high risk' DVTs.

PPL

- Limb elevation.
- Compression.
- Four-layer bandaging to achieve ulcer healing.
- Graduated compression stockings to maintain limb compression.
- (• Venous valve reconstruction.)

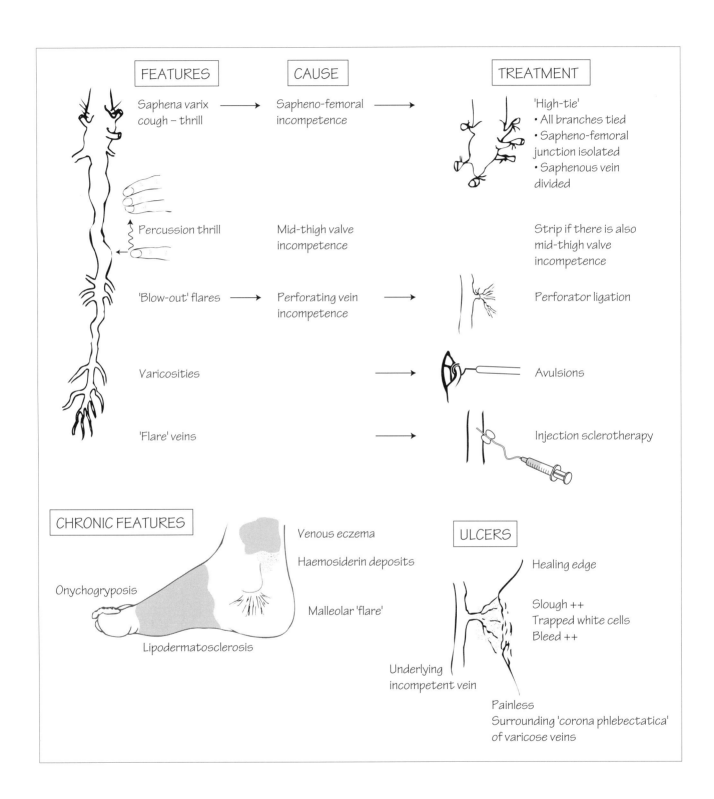

FEATURES

Saphena varix cough – thrill

Percussion thrill

'Blow-out' flares

Varicosities

'Flare' veins

CAUSE

Sapheno-femoral incompetence

Mid-thigh valve incompetence

Perforating vein incompetence

TREATMENT

'High-tie'
• All branches tied
• Sapheno-femoral junction isolated
• Saphenous vein divided

Strip if there is also mid-thigh valve incompetence

Perforator ligation

Avulsions

Injection sclerotherapy

CHRONIC FEATURES

Onychogryposis

Lipodermatosclerosis

Venous eczema

Haemosiderin deposits

Malleolar 'flare'

ULCERS

Healing edge

Slough ++
Trapped white cells
Bleed ++

Underlying incompetent vein

Painless
Surrounding 'corona phlebectatica' of varicose veins

Definition

Varicose veins are tortuous, dilated prominent superficial veins in the lower limbs, often in the anatomical distribution of the long and short saphenous veins.

KEY POINTS

- Surgery for varicose veins aims to divide all incompetent perforators and remove grossly diseased varicosities.
- Smaller varicose veins are best treated by injection sclerotherapy alone.
- Beware non-anatomical or atypical varicose veins in the young adult (congenital causes).
- Recurrent varicose veins require Duplex scanning assessment.

Epidemiology

Very common in the Western world, affecting about 50% of the adult population.

Aetiology

- Primary or familial varicose veins.
- Pregnancy (progesterone causes passive dilatation of veins).
- Secondary to postphlebitic limb (perforator failure).
- Congenital:
  Klippel–Trenaunay syndrome;
  Parkes–Weber syndrome.
- Iatrogenic: following formation of an arteriovenous fistula.

Pathophysiology

Venous valve failure, usually at the saphenofemoral junction (and sometimes in perforating veins), results in increased venous pressure in the long saphenous vein with progressive vein dilatation and further valve disruption.

Clinical features

- Asymptomatic.
- Cosmetic appearance.
- Dull aching leg pain. ⎤ Symptoms worse in the evening
- Heaviness in the leg. ⎦ or on standing for long periods.
- Itching and eczema.
- Superficial thrombophlebitis.
- Bleeding.
- Saphena varix.
- Ulceration.

Investigations

- Clinical assessment by Trendelenburg tourniquet tests.
- Doppler velocitometry: assess sapheno-femoral junction (SFJ)/short sapheno-popliteal junction (SSPJ).
- Duplex scanning: identify recurrence site (especially recurrent varicose veins).

ESSENTIAL MANAGEMENT

General

- Avoid long periods of standing.
- Elevate limbs.
- Wear support hosiery.

Specific

Injection sclerotherapy with sodium tetradecyl (STD)

- Suitable for small veins and usually only below the knee.
- Patients are encouraged to walk several miles per day.
- Anaphylaxis and local ulceration may occur.

Surgical ablation

- With the patient standing, the dilated veins are carefully marked with an indelible marker.
- The saphenous vein is surgically disconnected from the femoral vein and the perforators are also ablated.
- The elongated veins are removed via multiple stab incisions and long segments above the knee are removed using a 'vein stripper'.
- Postoperatively compression stockings are worn for several weeks and exercise is encouraged.
- Surgery is the most effective treatment for large varicose veins, but recurrence rates are high.

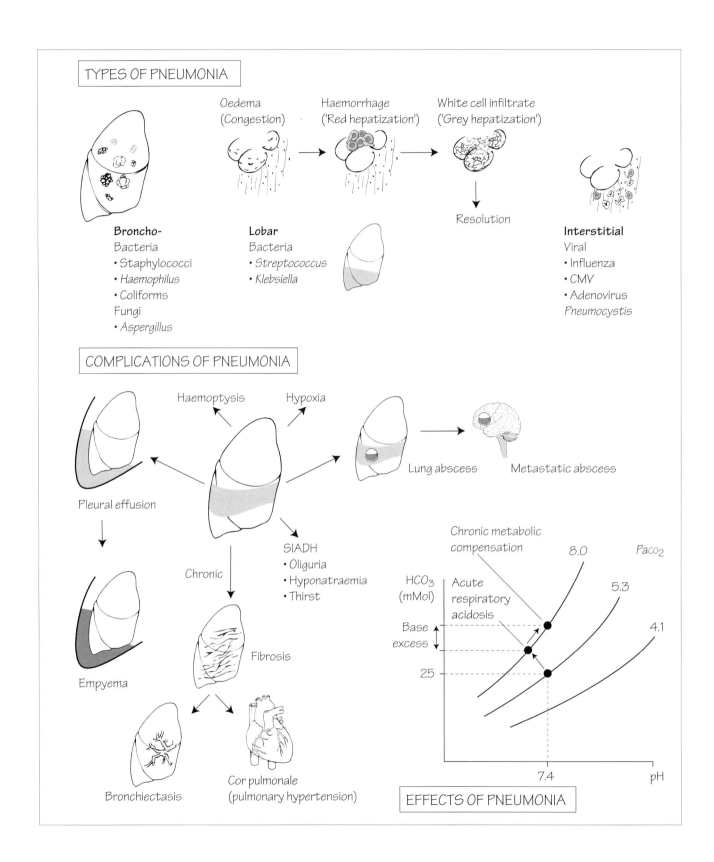

TYPES OF PNEUMONIA

Oedema (Congestion) → Haemorrhage ('Red hepatization') → White cell infiltrate ('Grey hepatization') → Resolution

Broncho-
Bacteria
• Staphylococci
• Haemophilus
• Coliforms
Fungi
• Aspergillus

Lobar
Bacteria
• Streptococcus
• Klebsiella

Interstitial
Viral
• Influenza
• CMV
• Adenovirus
Pneumocystis

COMPLICATIONS OF PNEUMONIA

Haemoptysis   Hypoxia

Lung abscess   Metastatic abscess

Pleural effusion

SIADH
• Oliguria
• Hyponatraemia
• Thirst

Chronic

Empyema

Fibrosis

Bronchiectasis   Cor pulmonale (pulmonary hypertension)

EFFECTS OF PNEUMONIA

Chronic metabolic compensation

HCO_3 (mMol)

Acute respiratory acidosis

Base excess

25

8.0   5.3   4.1 Pa_{CO_2}

7.4   pH

Definitions

Pulmonary collapse or *atelectasis* results from alveolar hypoventilation such that the alveolar walls collapse and become de-aerated. Pneumonia is an infection with consolidation of the pulmonary parenchyma.

> **KEY POINTS**
> - Thoracoabdominal incisions are at high risk of postoperative pulmonary collapse and infection.
> - Aggressive prophylaxis is key to prevention of complications.
> - Postoperative pneumonia is often due to mixed organisms.

Aetiology/pathophysiology

Postoperatively patients frequently develop atelectasis, which may develop into a pneumonia.

Pulmonary collapse
- Proximal bronchial obstruction.
- Trapped alveolar air absorbed.
- Common in smokers.
- Common with chronic bronchitis.

Pneumonia
- Infection with microorganisms.
- Bacterial: *Streptococcus pneumoniae, Staphylococcus, Haemophilus influenzae.*
- Viral: influenza, CMV.
- Fungal: *Candida, Aspergillus.*
- Protozoal: *Pneumocystis, Toxoplasma.*

Predisposing factors
- Secretional airway obstruction.
- Bronchorrhoea postsurgery.
- Mucus plugs block bronchi.
- Impaired ciliary action.
- Postoperative pain prevents effective coughing (especially thoracotomy and upper laparotomies).
- Organic airway obstruction.
- Bronchial neoplasm.

Patients prone to severe pneumonia
- The elderly.
- Alcoholics.
- Chronic lung and heart disease.
- Debilitated patients.
- Diabetes.
- Post-CVA.
- Immunodeficiency states.
- Postsplenectomy.
- Atelectasis postsurgery.

Clinical features

Pulmonary collapse
- Pyrexia.
- Tachypnoea.
- Diminished air entry.
- Bronchial breathing.

Pneumonia
- Respiratory distress.
- Painful dyspnoea.
- Tachypnoea.
- Productive cough ± haemoptysis.
- Hypoxia—confusion.
- Diminished air entry.
- Consolidation.
- Pleural rub.
- Cyanosis.

Investigations
- Chest X-ray: consolidation, pleural effusion, interstitial infiltrates, air-fluid cysts.
- Sputum culture: essential for correct antibiotic treatment.
- Blood gas analysis: diagnosis of respiratory failure.

ESSENTIAL MANAGEMENT

Prophylaxis
- Preoperative deep-breathing exercises.
- Incentive spirometry.
- Adequate analgesia postoperatively.
- Early ambulation.

Treatment
- Intensive chest physiotherapy.
- Respiratory support: humidified O_2 therapy; adequate hydration; bronchodilators if bronchospasm is present.
- Specific antimicrobial therapy.

Complications
- Respiratory failure.
- Lung abscess.

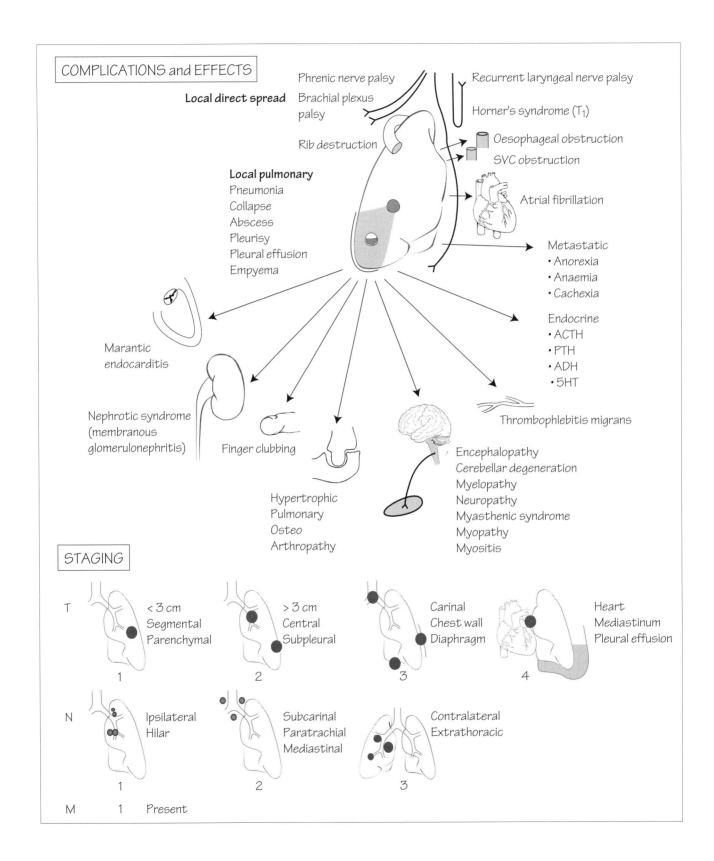

COMPLICATIONS and EFFECTS

Local direct spread

Phrenic nerve palsy

Brachial plexus palsy

Rib destruction

Recurrent laryngeal nerve palsy

Horner's syndrome (T_1)

Oesophageal obstruction

SVC obstruction

Atrial fibrillation

Local pulmonary
Pneumonia
Collapse
Abscess
Pleurisy
Pleural effusion
Empyema

Metastatic
• Anorexia
• Anaemia
• Cachexia

Endocrine
• ACTH
• PTH
• ADH
• 5HT

Marantic endocarditis

Nephrotic syndrome (membranous glomerulonephritis)

Finger clubbing

Hypertrophic Pulmonary Osteo Arthropathy

Thrombophlebitis migrans

Encephalopathy
Cerebellar degeneration
Myelopathy
Neuropathy
Myasthenic syndrome
Myopathy
Myositis

STAGING

T

< 3 cm
Segmental
Parenchymal

1

> 3 cm
Central
Subpleural

2

Carinal
Chest wall
Diaphragm

3

Heart
Mediastinum
Pleural effusion

4

N

Ipsilateral
Hilar

1

Subcarinal
Paratrachial
Mediastinal

2

Contralateral
Extrathoracic

3

M   1   Present

Definition

Malignant lesion of the respiratory tree epithelium.

> **KEY POINTS**
> - Symptoms may be masked by coexistent lung pathology (COPD).
> - Bronchial carcinoma often presents late and most are non-resectable.
> - Surgically resectable tumours have a fair prognosis.

Epidemiology

Male/female 5 : 1. Uncommon before 50 years. Most patients are in their 60s. Accounts for 40 000 deaths per annum in the UK.

Aetiology

The following are predisposing factors.
- Cigarette smoking.
- Air pollution.
- Exposure to uranium, chromium, arsenic, haematite and asbestos.

Pathology

Histology
- Squamous carcinoma: 50%.
- Small-cell (oat-cell) carcinoma: 35%.
- Adenocarcinoma: 15%.

Spread
- Direct to pleura, recurrent laryngeal nerve, pericardium, oesophagus, brachial plexus.
- Lymphatic to mediastinal and cervical nodes.
- Haematogenous to liver, bone, brain, adrenals.
- Transcoelomic pleural seedlings and effusion.

Clinical features

- History of tiredness, cough, anorexia, weight loss.
- Productive cough with purulent sputum.
- Haemoptysis.
- Finger clubbing.
- Bronchopneumonia (secondary infection of collapsed lung segment distal to malignant bronchial obstruction).
- Pleuritic pain.
- Neuropathy, myopathy, hypertrophic osteoarthropathy.
- Endocrine syndromes (ACTH is secreted by oat-cell tumours, parathormone is secreted by SCC—hypercalcaemia).
- Pancoast's tumour (apical tumour invading sympathetic trunk and brachial plexus)—Homer's syndrome, brachial neuralgia, paralysis of upper limb.
- Dysphagia and broncho-oesophageal fistula.
- Superior vena caval obstruction.

Investigations

Diagnostic
- Chest X-ray—PA and lateral (lung opacity, hilar lymphadenopathy).
- CT-guided lung biopsy.
- Sputum cytology.
- Bronchoscopy and cytology of brushings or lavage fluid.

Assess operability
- Helical CT scan of thorax/abdomen: involvement of adjacent structures, hepatic metastases, multiple primary lesions.
- Bone scan: metastases.
- Liver ultrasound: metastases.
- Mediastinoscopy: involvement of mediastinal nodes.
- Lung function test: likely patient tolerance of pulmonary resection.

ESSENTIAL MANAGEMENT

Surgical
- Indicated only for non-small cell tumours when tumour is confined to one lobe or lung, no evidence of secondary deposits, carina is tumour free on bronchoscopy.
- Operation: lobectomy or pneumonectomy.

Palliative

Radiotherapy (small-cell carcinoma most radiosensitive): stop haemoptysis, relieve bone pain from secondaries, relieve superior vena caval obstruction.

Prognosis

Following 'curative' resection 5-year survival rates are approximately 20–30%, but overall 5-year survival is only about 6%.

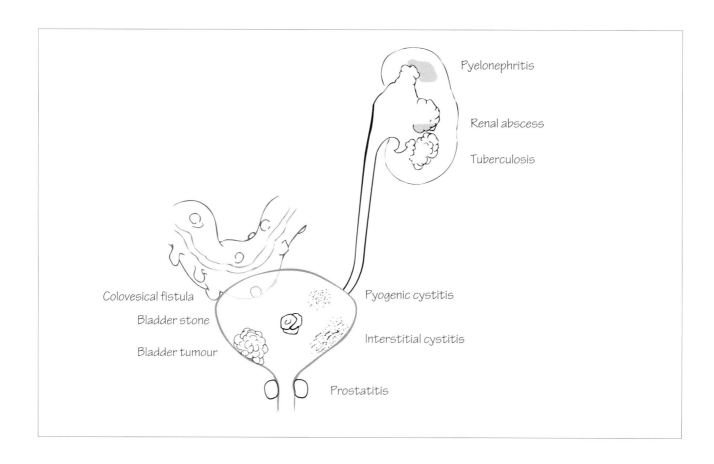

Definitions

A *urinary tract infection* (UTI) is a documented episode of significant bacteriuria (i.e. an infection with a colony count of >100 000 single organisms per ml) which may affect the upper (*pyelonephritis*, *renal abscess*) or the lower (*cystitis*) urinary tract or both.

> **KEY POINTS**
> - Lower UTI is usually harmless and simple to treat.
> - Upper UTI may be associated with renal damage and major complications and requires prompt investigation and treatment.
> - Consider an underlying cause in all recurrent or atypical infections.

Epidemiology

UTI is a very common condition in general practice (usually *Escherichia coli*) and accounts for 40% of hospital-acquired (*nosocomial*) infections (often *Enterobacter* or *Klebsiella*).

Risk factors

- Urinary tract obstruction.
- Instrumentation of urinary tract (e.g. indwelling catheter).
- Dysfunctional (neuropathic) bladder.
- Immunosuppression.
- Diabetes mellitus.
- Structural abnormalities (e.g. vesicoureteric reflux).
- Pregnancy.

Pathology

- Ascending infection: most UTIs caused in this way (bacteria from GI tract colonize lower urinary tract).
- Haematogenous spread: infrequent cause of UTI (seen in i.v. drug users, bacterial endocarditis and TB).

Clinical features

Upper urinary tract infection

- Fever, rigors/chill.
- Flank pain.
- Malaise.
- Anorexia.
- Costovertebral angle and abdominal tenderness.

Lower urinary tract infection

- Dysuria.
- Frequency and urgency.
- Suprapubic pain.
- Haematuria.
- Scrotal pain (epididymo-orchitis) or perineal pain (prostatitis).

Investigations

Gram stain and culture of a 'clean-catch' urine specimen before antibiotics have been given. Usual organisms are *E. coli*, *Enterobacter*, *Klebsiella*, *Proteus* (suggests presence of urinary calculi).

Upper urinary tract infection

- FBC.
- U+E and serum creatinine: renal function.
- Renal ultrasound: swelling in pyelonephritis, stones, obstruction/hydronephrosis, secondary abscess.
- IVU: stones, structural abnormalities, obstructed collecting system.
- CT scan: abscess/tumours.
- Isotope scan (DPTA, DMSA): renal tubuloglomerular function.

Lower urinary tract infection

- FBC.
- Cystoscopy only if haematuria—underlying neoplasm or stones.
- If obstruction is present ultrasound scan, IVU and cystoscopy may be needed.

> **ESSENTIAL MANAGEMENT**
> Treat the infection with an appropriate antibiotic based on urine culture results and deal with any underlying cause (e.g. relieve obstruction). High fluid intake should be encouraged and potassium citrate may relieve dysuria.
>
> **Upper tract UTIs, epididymo-orchitis and prostatitis**
> - i.v. antibiotic therapy (ciprofloxacin, gentamicin, cefuroxime, co-trimoxazole).
> - Relieve acute obstruction with internal (stent) or external (nephrostomy) drainage (especially if acute severe sepsis).
> - An abscess will require drainage either radiologically or surgically.
>
> **Cystitis and uncomplicated lower UTI**
> - Oral antibiotics (trimethoprim, ciprofloxacin, nitrofurantoin, cephradine).
> - If there is a poor response to treatment consider unusual urinary infections: tuberculosis (sterile pyuria), candiduria, schistosomiasis, *Chlamydia trachomatis*, *Neisseria gonorrhoeae*.
> - Recurrent infections should raise the possibility of underlying abnormalities requiring investigation.

Complications

- Bacteraemia and septic shock.
- Renal, perinephric and metastatic abscesses.
- Renal damage and acute/chronic renal failure.
- Chronic and xanthogranulomatous pyelonephritis.

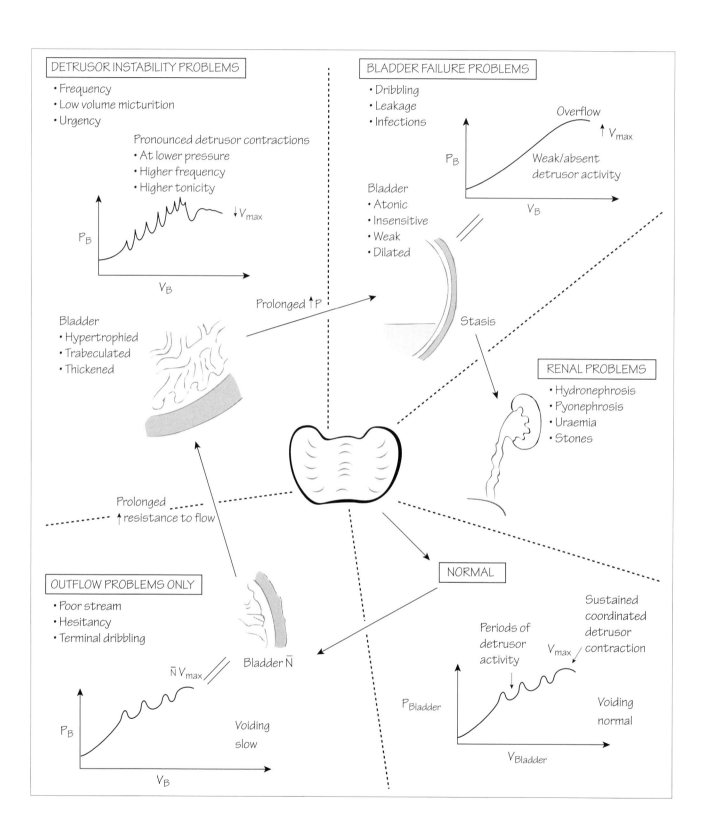

DETRUSOR INSTABILITY PROBLEMS
- Frequency
- Low volume micturition
- Urgency

Pronounced detrusor contractions
- At lower pressure
- Higher frequency
- Higher tonicity

$\downarrow V_{max}$

P_B

V_B

Bladder
- Hypertrophied
- Trabeculated
- Thickened

Prolonged $\uparrow P$

BLADDER FAILURE PROBLEMS
- Dribbling
- Leakage
- Infections

Overflow

$\uparrow V_{max}$

P_B

Weak/absent detrusor activity

V_B

Bladder
- Atonic
- Insensitive
- Weak
- Dilated

Stasis

RENAL PROBLEMS
- Hydronephrosis
- Pyonephrosis
- Uraemia
- Stones

Prolonged $\uparrow$ resistance to flow

OUTFLOW PROBLEMS ONLY
- Poor stream
- Hesitancy
- Terminal dribbling

$\bar{N} V_{max}$

P_B

V_B

Bladder $\bar{N}$

Voiding slow

NORMAL

Periods of detrusor activity

Sustained coordinated detrusor contraction

V_{max}

$P_{Bladder}$

Voiding normal

$V_{Bladder}$

Definition

Benign prostatic hypertrophy (BPH) is a condition of unknown aetiology characterized by an increase in size of the inner zone (periurethral glands) of the prostate gland.

> **KEY POINTS**
> • Symptoms of BPH are initially due to outflow problems, then bladder instability, then bladder failure.
> • Early treatment of symptoms prevents/reverses bladder damage and complications.
> • Surgical resection is safe but is associated with some significant complications.

Epidemiology

Present in 50% of 60–90-year-old-men.

Pathophysiology

• Microscopic stromal nodules develop around the periurethral glands.
• Glandular hyperplasia originates around these nodules.
• As the gland increases in size, it compresses the urethra, leading to urinary tract obstruction.

Clinical features

Initially outlet obstruction:
• Weak stream, hesitancy, intermittency, dribbling, straining to void, acute urinary retention.
Subsequent detrusor instability:
• Frequency, urgency, nocturia, dysuria, urge incontinence.
Finally detrusor failure and chronic retention:
• Palpable (or percussible) bladder, overflow incontinence.
• Enlarged smooth prostate on digital rectal examination.

Investigations

Basic investigations

• Urinalysis and urine culture for evidence of infection or haematuria.
• FBC: infection.
• U+E and serum creatinine: renal function.
• PSA: suspicion of underlying malignancy.

Further investigations

• Voiding diary.
• Uroflowmetry and residual volume measurement (normal <100 ml): evidence of obstruction.
• Ultrasonography of kidneys and bladder: structural abnormalities.
• Transrectal ultrasound: to determine prostate size.
• IVU: structural abnormalities.
• Cystoscopy.

ESSENTIAL MANAGEMENT

Medical
• Alter oral fluid intake, reduce caffeine intake.
• α-Adrenergic blockers (e.g. phenoxybenzamine, prazosin).
• Anti-androgens acting selectively at prostatic cellular level (e.g. finasteride).
• Intermittent self-catheterization if detrusor failure.
• Balloon dilatation and stenting of prostate (unfit patient).

Surgical
• Majority of patients are treated surgically.
• Surgical removal of the adenomatous portion of the prostate.
• TURP with electrocautery or laser.
• Thermal ablation of prostate.
• Open prostatectomy if large which may be transvesical or retropubic.

Complications of surgical treatment

• Postoperative haemorrhage and clot retention.
• UTI.
• Retrograde ejaculation, impotence.
• TURP syndrome: in 2% of patients absorption of irrigation fluid via venous sinuses in the prostate causes hyponatraemia, hypotension and metabolic acidosis.
• Incontinence.
• Urethral stricture.

Prognosis

The majority of patients have a very good quality of life after prostatectomy (endoscopic or open).

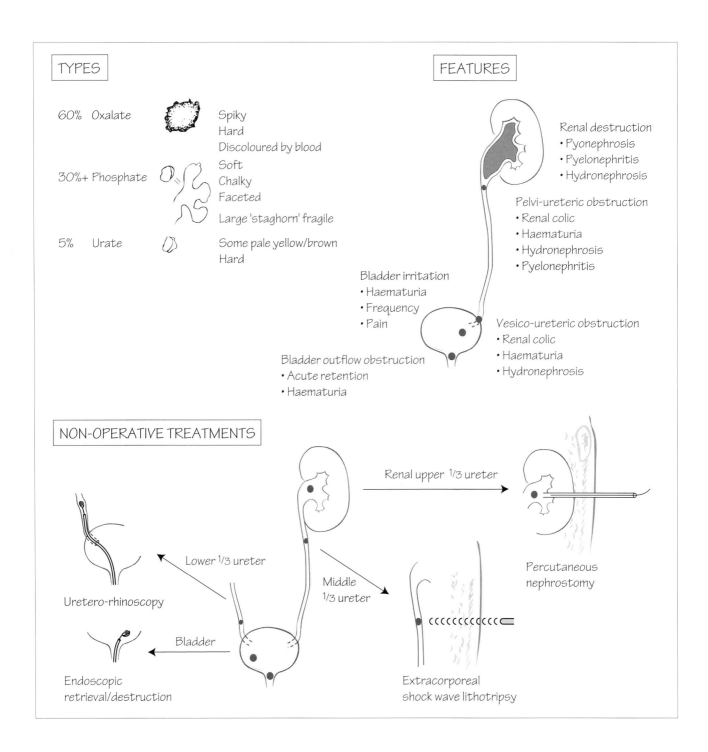

TYPES

60%   Oxalate — Spiky / Hard / Discoloured by blood

30%+ Phosphate — Soft / Chalky / Faceted / Large 'staghorn' fragile

5%   Urate — Some pale yellow/brown / Hard

FEATURES

Renal destruction
• Pyonephrosis
• Pyelonephritis
• Hydronephrosis

Pelvi-ureteric obstruction
• Renal colic
• Haematuria
• Hydronephrosis
• Pyelonephritis

Bladder irritation
• Haematuria
• Frequency
• Pain

Vesico-ureteric obstruction
• Renal colic
• Haematuria
• Hydronephrosis

Bladder outflow obstruction
• Acute retention
• Haematuria

NON-OPERATIVE TREATMENTS

Renal upper 1/3 ureter

Lower 1/3 ureter

Middle 1/3 ureter

Bladder

Uretero-rhinoscopy

Endoscopic retrieval/destruction

Extracorporeal shock wave lithotripsy

Percutaneous nephrostomy

Definition

Renal calculi are concretions formed by precipitation of various urinary solutes in the urinary tract. They contain calcium oxalate (60%), phosphate as a mixture of calcium, ammonium and magnesium phosphate (triple phosphate stones are infective in origin) (30%), uric acid (5%) and cystine (1%).

> **KEY POINTS**
> - Calculi may develop because of or cause UTIs.
> - Most stones pass without complication.
> - Most stones are managed non-surgically.

Epidemiology

Male > female. Early adult life. Among Europeans prevalence is 3%.

Pathogenesis

- Hypercalciuria: 65% of patients have idiopathic hypercalciuria.
- Nucleation theory: a crystal or foreign body acts as a nucleus for crystallization of supersaturated urine.
- Stone matrix theory: a protein matrix secreted by renal tubular cells acts as a scaffold for crystallization of supersaturated urine.
- Reduced inhibition theory: reduced urinary levels of naturally occurring inhibitors of crystallization.
- Dehydration.
- Infection: staghorn triple phosphate calculi are formed by the action of urease-producing organisms (*Proteus*, *Klebsiella*), which produce ammonia and render the urine alkaline. Schistosomiasis predisposes to bladder calculi (and cancer).

Pathology

- Staghorn calculi are large, fill the renal pelvis and calices, and lead to recurring pyelonephritis and renal parenchymal damage.
- Other stones are smaller, ranging in size from a few millimetres to 1–2 cm. They cause problems by obstructing the urinary tract, usually the ureter. Calyceal stones may cause haematuria and bladder stones may cause infection. Chronic bladder stones predispose to the unusual squamous carcinoma of the bladder.

Clinical features

- Calyceal stones may be asymptomatic.
- Staghorn calculi present with loin pain and upper-tract UTI.
- Ureteric colic—severe colicky pain radiating from the loin to the groin and into the testes or labia associated with gross or microscopic haematuria.
- Bladder calculi present with sudden interruption of urinary stream, perineal pain and pain at the tip of the penis.

Investigations

- FBC, U+E, serum creatinine, calcium, phosphate, urate, proteins and alkaline phosphatase.
- Urine microscopy for haematuria and crystals.
- Urine culture: secondary infection.
- Plain abdominal X-ray: 90% of renal calculi are radio-opaque.
- IVU: confirms the presence and identifies the position of the stone in the genito-urinary tract.
- A renogram: may be indicated with staghorn calculi to assess renal function.
- 24-hour urine collection when patient is at home in normal environment.
- Stone analysis: origin.

> **ESSENTIAL MANAGEMENT**
> - Pain relief for ureteric colic: pethidine, diclofenac. High fluid intake.
> - 80% of ureteric stones pass spontaneously. Stones of <4 mm in diameter almost always pass, >6 mm almost never pass.
> - Indications for intervention:
>   kidney stones: symptomatic, obstruction, staghorn;
>   ureteric stones: failure to pass, large stone, obstruction, infection;
>   bladder stones: all to prevent complications;
>   sepsis super-added: nephrostomy.

Interventional procedures

- ESWL for small/medium kidney stones.
- Percutaneous nephrolithotomy for large kidney stones and staghorn calculi.
- ESWL or contact lithotrypsy for upper ureteric stones (above pelvic brim).
- Contact lithotrypsy or extraction with a Dormia basket for lower ureteric stones.
- Open surgery: ureterolithotomy or nephrolithotomy.
- Mechanical lithotrypsy or open surgery for bladder stones.

73 Renal cell carcinoma

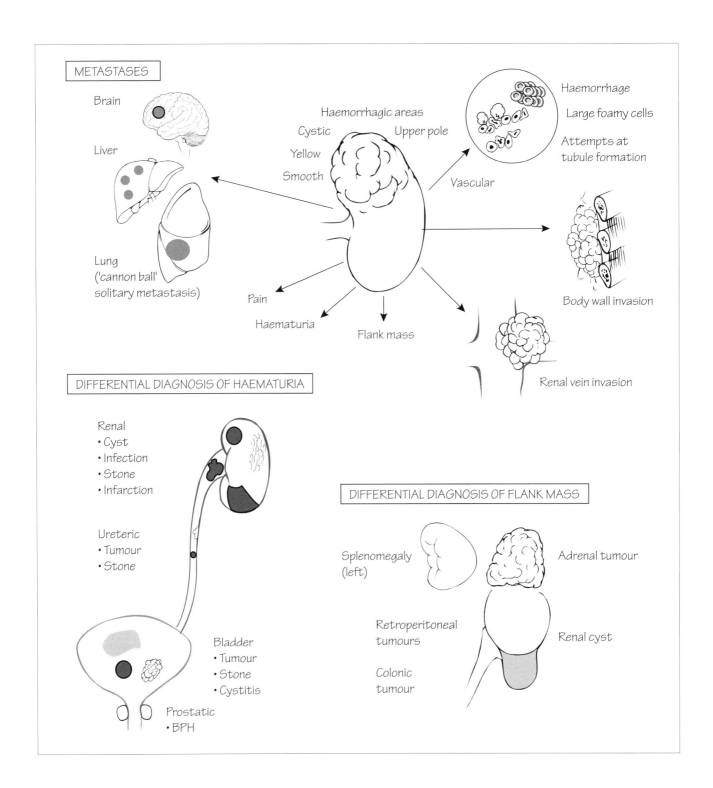

Definitions

Malignant lesion (*adenocarcinoma*) of the kidney epithelium (also known as *hypernephroma* and *Grawitz tumour*).

> **KEY POINTS**
> - New, significant haematuria always requires investigation and may represent renal cell carcinoma (RCC).
> - Consider RCC in unexplained anaemia, vague abdominal symptoms and recurrent UTIs.
> - Surgery offers the best hope of long-term survival.
> - Tumours are occasionally familial and a family history should be sought.

Epidemiology

Male/female 2 : 1. Uncommon before 40 years. Accounts for 2–3% of all tumours in adults and 85% of all renal tumours. (The other renal tumours are urothelial tumours, Wilms' tumour and sarcomas.)

Aetiology

Predisposing factors

- Diet: high intake of fat, oil and milk.
- Toxic agents: lead, cadmium, asbestos, petroleum by-products.
- Smoking.
- Genetic factors: oncogene on short arm of chromosome 3, HLA antigen BW-44 and DR-8.
- Other diseases: von Hippel–Lindau (VHL) syndrome, adult polycystic disease, renal dialysis patients.

Pathology

Histology

Adenocarcinoma (cell of origin is the proximal convoluted tubular cell).

Staging

- TNM staging.
- Robson stages I–IV
  Stage I: tumour confined within renal capsule.
  Stage II: tumour confined by Gerota's fascia.
  Stage III: tumour to renal vein or IVC, nodes or through Gerota's fascia.
  Stage IV: distant metastases or invasion of adjacent organs.

Spread

- Direct into renal vein and perirenal tissue.
- Lymphatic to periaortic and hilar nodes.
- Haematogenous to lung (large, 'cannon-ball' metastases), bones and contralateral kidney.

Clinical features

- Triad of haematuria (50–60%), flank pain (35–50%), palpable abdominal mass (25–45%). All three are present in <10% of patients.
- Hypertension, polycythaemia (due to decreased blood flow to JGA → ↑renin, ↑erythropoietin).
- Anaemia, weight loss, PUO.
- Hypercalcaemia, ectopic hormone production (ACTH, ADH).
- Liver dysfunction (raised enzymes and prolonged PT) in the absence of metastatic disease.
- Renal carcinoma is one of the 'great mimics' of medicine.

Investigations

- FBC: anaemia, polycythaemia.
- ESR.
- U+E, creatinine: renal function.
- LFTs: metastases.
- Urine culture: infection.
- Abdominal ultrasound: assess renal mass and IVC.
- Helical CT scan: assess renal mass, fixity, nodes.
- IVU: image renal outline.
- Cavagram and echocardiogram: assess IVC and right atrium involvement.

> **ESSENTIAL MANAGEMENT**
> **Surgical**
> - Offers best chance of long-term survival.
> - Partial: if Stage I and part of VHL presentation.
> - Radical: aim to remove kidney, renal vessels, upper ureter, adrenal and Gerota's fascia.
> - Isolated lung metastases may also be removed surgically with good results.
>
> **Palliative**
> - Renal artery embolization (may stop haematuria).
> - Chemotherapy (only 10% response rate).
> - Hormone therapy (only 5% response rate).
> - Immunotherapy (currently under review).

Prognosis

Overall survival is 40% at 5 years.

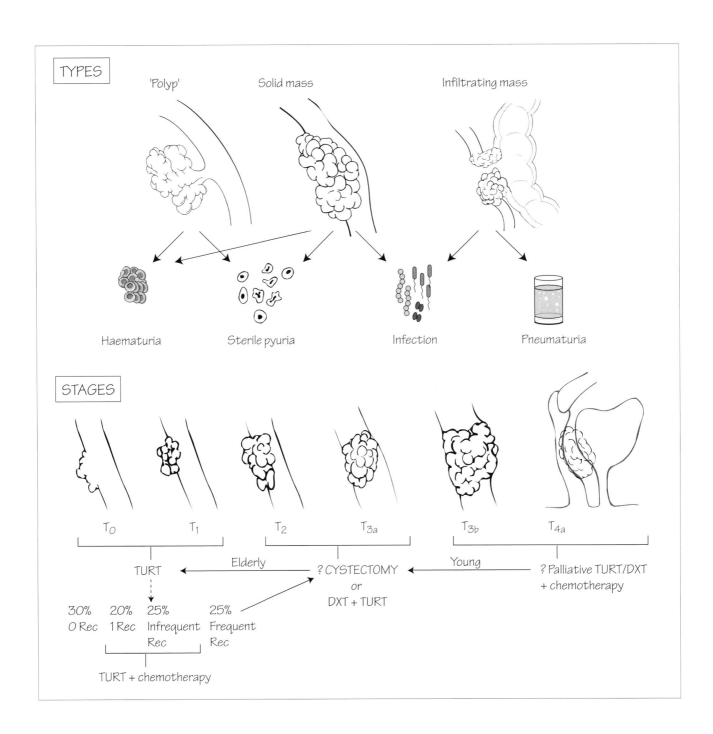

Definition

Malignant lesion of the bladder epithelium.

> **KEY POINTS**
> - Commonly presents with haematuria.
> - Ranges from 'benign' acting recurrent bladder 'polyps' to rapidly progressive infiltrating masses.
> - Transitional cell lesions are a 'field' change and often multiple.

Epidemiology

Male > female. Uncommon before 50 years. Increasing incidence of bladder cancer in recent years. Death rate is 7.6/100 000.

Aetiology

Predisposing factors:
- Exposure to carcinogens in rubber industry (1- and 2-naphthylamine, benzidine, aminobiphenyl).
- Smoking, tryptophan metabolites, phenacitan.
- Bladder schistosomiasis, and chronic bladder stones (squamous carcinoma).
- Congenital abnormalities (extrophy of the bladder) (adenocarcinoma).

Pathology

Histology

- Transitional cell carcinoma (TCC).
- Squamous cell carcinoma (rare).
- Adenocarcinoma (rare).

Staging for TCC

	T_{IS}	Carcinoma *in situ*
Superficial tumours	T_a	Tumour confined to urothelium
	T_1	Lamina propria involved
Invasive tumours	T_2	Superficial muscle invasion
	T_{3a}	Deep muscle invasion
	T_{3b}	Serosal involvement
Fixed tumours	T_{4a}	Invasion of prostate, uterus or vagina
	T_{4b}	Fixation to pelvic wall

Spread

- Direct into pelvic viscera (prostate, uterus, vagina, colon, rectum).
- Lymphatic to periaortic nodes.
- Haematogenous to liver and lung.

Clinical features

- Painless intermittent haematuria (95%).
- Dysuria or frequency (10%).

Investigations

- Urine cytology.
- IVU: occult upper tract tumours.
- Cystourethroscopy.
- FBC: anaemia.
- U+E creatinine: renal function.
- Ultrasound: obstruction.
- CT scan: local invasion, distant metastases.

> **ESSENTIAL MANAGEMENT**
>
> **Carcinoma *in situ* (T_{IS})**
> - Intravesical chemotherapy for isolated carcinoma-*in-situ* and associated with papillary tumours.
> - Cystourethrectomy for unresponsive lesions and 'malignant' cystitis.
>
> **Superficial tumours (T_a, T_1)**
> - TURT and follow-up cystoscopy.
> - If recurrences or increased risk of invasion (large tumours, multiple tumours, severe dysplasia or carcinoma-*in-situ*) intravesical chemotherapy (mitomycin-C, BCG).
> - Persistent recurrences despite therapy—cystourethrectomy.
>
> **Invasive tumours (T_2, T_3)**
> - TURT + radical radiotherapy; or
> - Radical cystectomy (and reconstruction or urinary diversion, e.g. by ileal conduit).
>
> **Fixed tumours (T_4)**
> - Chemotherapy: MVAC (methotrexate, vinblastine, adriamycin, cisplatin), CMV (cisplatin, methotrexate, vinblastine), Cisca (cisplatin, cyclophosphamide, adriamycin).
> - Radiotherapy and TURT for palliation.

Prognosis

- Superficial tumours: 75% 5-year survival.
- Invasive tumours: 10% 5-year survival.
- Fixed tumours and metastases: median survival 1 year.
- Long-term follow-up required for life.

75 Carcinoma of the prostate

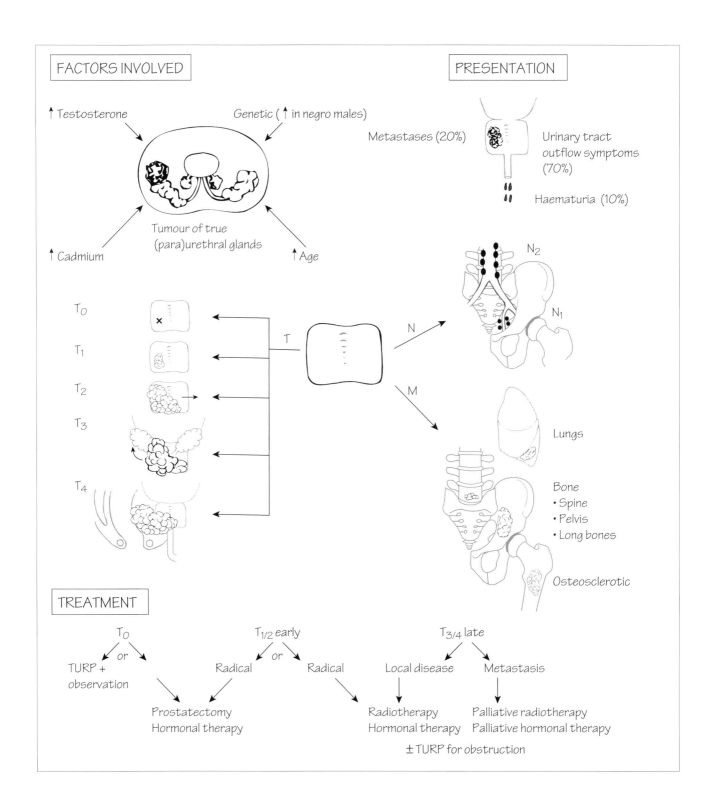

Definition

Malignant lesion of the prostate gland.

KEY POINTS
- Prostatic cancer is common and should be considered in all new symptoms of lower urinary tract obstruction.
- Increasingly found (asymptomatic) by screening.
- Early treatment offers good 5-year survival with combined surgery and hormonal adjuvants.
- Late presentation disease is best managed medically and has a poor outlook.

Epidemiology

Uncommon before 60 years. 80% of prostate cancers are clinically undetected (latent carcinoma) and are only discovered on autopsy. The true incidence of this disease is considerably higher than the clinical experience would indicate.

Aetiology

- Increasing age.
- More common in negro males.
- Hormonal factors: prostate cancer growth is enhanced by testosterone and inhibited by oestrogens or antiandrogens.

Pathology

Prostatic tumours are often multicentric and located in the periphery of the gland.

Histology

- Adenocarcinoma arising from glandular epithelium.
- Gleason grading (1–5) is used to grade differentiation.

Staging

	T_0	Unsuspected
Localized	T_1	Histological diagnosis only (clinical, radiology –ve)
	T_2	Palpable—confined within prostate
Local spread	T_3	Spread to seminal vesicles
	T_4	Spread to pelvic wall
	T_{1-4}, M_1	Metastatic disease

Spread

- Direct into remainder of gland and seminal vesicles.
- Lymphatic to iliac and periaortic nodes.
- Haematogenous to bone (usually osteosclerotic lesions), liver, lung.

Clinical features

- Bladder outflow obstruction (poor stream, hesitancy, nocturia).
- Symptoms of advanced disease (ureteric obstruction and hydronephrosis or bone pain from metastases, classically worse at night).
- Nodule or mass detected on rectal examination.

Investigations

- FBC: anaemia.
- U+E, creatinine: renal function.
- Specific markers: PSA, alkaline and acid phosphatase.
- Transrectal ultrasound and MRI: local staging.
- Needle biopsy of the prostate: tissue diagnosis.
- Bone scan: metastases.

ESSENTIAL MANAGEMENT
- T_0: observation, repeated digital (or ultrasound) examination and PSA.
- T_{1+2}: radical prostatectomy or radical radiotherapy, or interstitial radiation with ^{125}I or ^{198}Au.
- T_{3+4}: external beam radiation $\pm$ hormonal therapy.
- Metastatic: hormonal manipulation, bilateral orchidectomy, stilboestrol, LH-RH agonists, antiandrogens (cyproterone acetate), radiotherapy and strontium for bony metastases.

Prognosis

- Localized tumours: 80% 5-year survival.
- Local spread: 40% 5-year survival.
- Metastases: 20% 5-year survival.

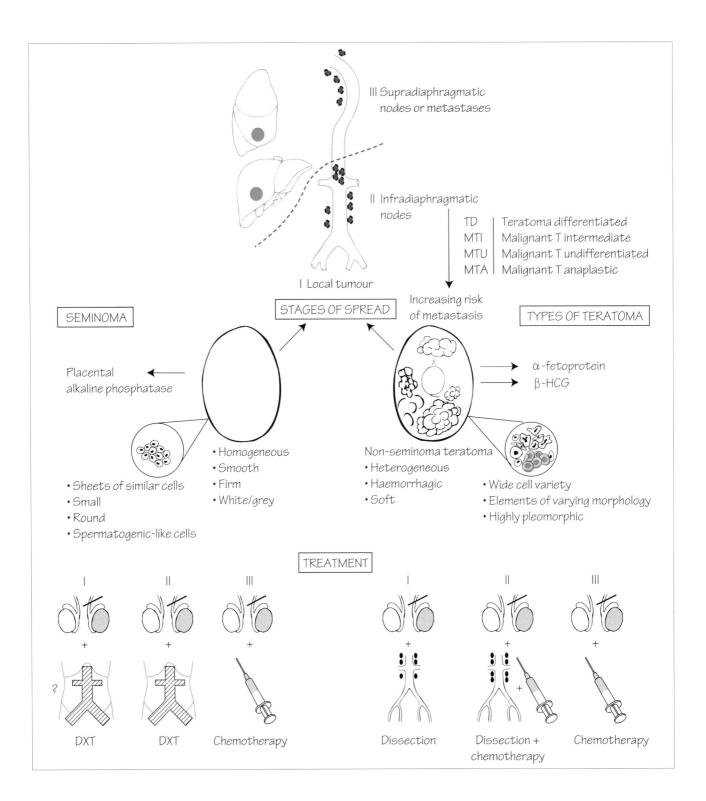

Definition
Malignant lesion of the testis.

Epidemiology
Age 20–40 years. Commonest solid tumours in young males.

Aetiology
- Cryptorchidism—50-fold increase in risk of developing testicular cancer. Risk is unaffected by orchidopexy.
- Higher incidence in white men.

Pathology
Classification of testicular tumours
- Germ-cell tumours (90%) (secrete AFP and (β-HCG)):
  seminoma;
  non-seminoma—embryonal carcinoma, teratocarcinoma, choriocarcinoma.
- Stromal tumours:
  Leydig cell;
  Sertoli cell;
  granulosa cell.
- Metastatic tumours.

Staging
- Stage I: confined to scrotum.
- Stage II: spread to retroperitoneal lymph nodes below the diaphragm.
- Stage III: distant metastases.

Spread
- Germ-cell tumours metastasize to the para-aortic nodes, lung and brain.
- Stromal tumours rarely metastasize.

Clinical features
- Painless swelling of the testis, often discovered incidentally or after trauma.
- Vague testicular discomfort common, bleeding into tumour may mimic acute torsion.
- Rarely evidence of metastatic disease or gynaecomastia.
- Examination reveals a hard, irregular, non-tender testicular mass.

Investigations
- Blood for tumour markers, i.e. AFP and β-HCG.
- AFP is elevated in 75% of embryonal and 65% of teratocarcinoma.
- AFP is not elevated in pure seminoma or choriocarcinoma.
- β-HCG is elevated in 100% choriocarcinoma, 60% embryonal carcinoma, 60% teratocarcinoma and 10% pure seminoma.
- Scrotal ultrasound: diagnosis.
- Chest X-ray to assess lungs and mediastinum: metastases.
- CT scan of chest and abdomen: to detect lymph nodes.
- Laparoscopy (retroperitoneoscopy): to assess abdominal nodes.

ESSENTIAL MANAGEMENT
Radical orchidectomy (via groin incision) and histological diagnosis. Further treatment depends on histology and staging.

Seminoma
- Stage I: radiotherapy to abdominal nodes.
- Stage II: radiotherapy to abdominal nodes.
- Stage III: chemotherapy (bleomycin, etoposide, cisplatin).

Non-seminoma germ cell
- Stage 1: Retroperitoneal lymph node dissection (RPLND).
- Stage II: chemotherapy + RPLND.
- Stage III: chemotherapy (+ RPLND if good response).

Prognosis
Overall cure rates are over 90% and node-negative disease has almost 100% 5-year survival.

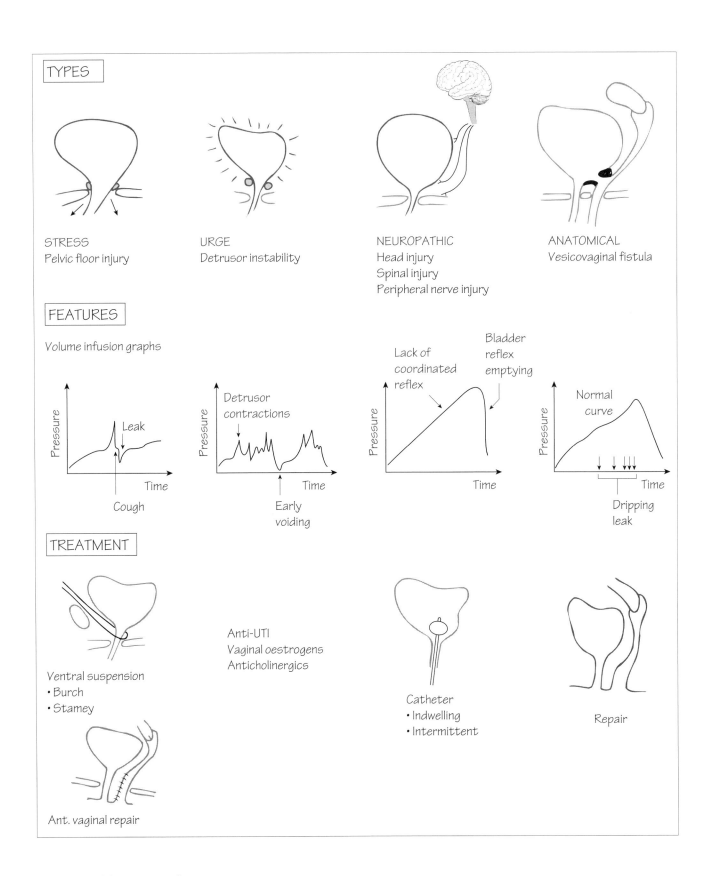

TYPES

STRESS
Pelvic floor injury

URGE
Detrusor instability

NEUROPATHIC
Head injury
Spinal injury
Peripheral nerve injury

ANATOMICAL
Vesicovaginal fistula

FEATURES

Volume infusion graphs

Leak
Cough

Detrusor contractions
Early voiding

Lack of coordinated reflex
Bladder reflex emptying

Normal curve
Dripping leak

TREATMENT

Ventral suspension
• Burch
• Stamey

Ant. vaginal repair

Anti-UTI
Vaginal oestrogens
Anticholinergics

Catheter
• Indwelling
• Intermittent

Repair

Definition

Urinary incontinence is defined as the involuntary loss of urine.

> **KEY POINTS**
> * A common and socially disabling condition.
> * Full assessment and investigation is required to elicit precise cause and tailor treatment properly.
> * Always assess if bladder full or empty (overflow or otherwise).

Physiology

Normal bladder capacity is 350–400 ml. As the bladder fills with urine, the detrusor muscle relaxes to accommodate the rise in volume without a rise in pressure (plasticity). When the bladder is full, stretch receptors in the bladder wall initiate a reflex contraction (via S3,4) of the detrusor muscle and relaxation of the urinary sphincter to empty the bladder. This spinal reflex is controlled by an inhibitory cortical mechanism, which allows conscious control over micturition. Conscious control develops during early childhood.

Classification

Urethral incontinence

* Urethral abnormalities: obesity, multiparity, difficult delivery, pelvic fractures, postprostatectomy.
* Bladder abnormalities: neuropathic or non-neuropathic detrusor abnormalities, infection, interstitial cystitis, bladder stones and tumours.
* Non-urinary abnormalities: impaired mobility or mental function.

Non-urethral incontinence

* Urinary fistula: vesicovaginal.
* Ureteral ectopia: ureter drains into urethra (usually a duplex ureter).

Pathophysiology

* *Stress incontinence*: urine leakage occurs when infra-abdominal pressure exceeds urethral pressure (e.g. coughing, straining or lifting), usually in the presence of urethral incompetence.
* *Urge incontinence*: idiopathic detrusor instability causes a rise in intravesical pressure and urine leakage.
* *Detrusor hyperreflexia*: loss of cortical control results in an uninhibited bladder with unstable detrusor contractions. The bladder fills, the sacral reflex is initiated and the bladder empties spontaneously.
* *Overflow incontinence*: damage to the efferent fibres of the sacral reflex causes bladder atonia. The bladder fills with urine and becomes grossly distended with constant dribbling of urine, e.g. chronic bladder distension from obstruction.

Clinical features

* Stress incontinence: loss of urine during coughing, straining, etc. These symptoms are quite specific for stress incontinence.
* Urge incontinence: inability to maintain urine continence in the presence of frequent and insistent urges to void.
* Nocturnal enuresis: 10% of 5-year-olds and 5% of 10-year-olds are incontinent during sleep. Bed wetting in older children is abnormal and may indicate the presence of an unstable bladder.
* Symptoms of urinary infection (frequency, dysuria, nocturia), obstruction (poor stream, dribbling), trauma (including surgery, e.g. abdominoperineal resection), fistula (continuous dribbling), neurological disease (sexual or bowel dysfunction) or systemic disease (e.g. diabetes) may point to an underlying cause.

Investigations

* Urine culture: to exclude infection.
* IVU: to assess upper tracts and obstruction or fistula.
* Urodynamics:
  uroflowmetry: measures flow rate;
  cystometry: demonstrates detrusor contractures;
  video cystometry: shows leakage of urine on straining in patients with stress incontinence;
  urethral pressure flowmetry: measures urethral and bladder pressure at rest and during voiding.
* Cystoscopy: if bladder stone or neoplasm is suspected.
* Vaginal speculum examination ± cystogram if vesicovaginal fistula suspected.

ESSENTIAL MANAGEMENT

Urge incontinence
* Medical treatment: modify fluid intake, avoid caffeine, treat any underlying cause (infection, tumour, stone); bladder training; anticholinergic/smooth muscle relaxants (oxybutinin, tolterdine).
* Surgical treatment: cystoscopy and bladder distension, augmentation cystoplasty.

Stress incontinence
* Medical treatment: pelvic floor exercises, oestrogens for atrophic vaginitis.
* Surgical treatment: retropubic or endoscopic urethropexy, vaginal repair, artificial sphincter.

Overflow incontinence
* If obstruction present: treat cause of obstruction, e.g. TURP.
* If no obstruction: short period of catheter drainage to allow detrusor muscle to recover from overstretching, then short course of detrusor muscle stimulants (bethanehol; distigmine). If all else fails, clean intermittent self-catheterization (neurogenic overflow incontinence).

Urinary fistula
Always requires surgical treatment.

Gastro-oesophageal reflux
Definition
This is a common condition characterized by incompetence of the lower oesophageal sphincter, resulting in retrograde passage of gastric contents into the oesophagus, leading to vomiting.

Aetiology
Immaturity of lower oesophageal sphincter; short intra-abdominal oesophagus.

Clinical features
• Vomiting, usually bile-stained, not related to feeds, may contain blood (indicates oesophagitis) and rarely is projectile.
• Failure to thrive may indicate repeated episodes of aspiration and pneumonia.

Investigation
If oesophagitis, stricture, anaemia or aspiration is suspected, a barium swallow, oesophagoscopy and biopsy, 24-hour pH monitoring and oesophageal manometry are indicated.

Treatment
• As there is a natural tendency towards spontaneous improvement with age, a conservative approach is adopted initially: thickening of feeds, positioning infant in 30° head-up prone position after feeds, antacids (e.g. Gaviscon®), drugs to increase gastric emptying and increase lower oesophageal sphincter tone (e.g. Cisapride®).
• Surgery (laparoscopic Nissen fundoplication) is reserved for failure for respond to conservative treatment with oesophageal stricture or severe pulmonary aspiration.

Infantile hypertrophic pyloric stenosis
Definition
This is a condition characterized by hypertrophy of the circular muscle of the gastric pylorus that obstructs gastric outflow.

Aetiology
The aetiology is unknown but it affects 1 : 450 children; 85% male, often firstborn; 20% have family history.

Clinical features
• Non-bile-stained, projectile vomiting (after feeds) beginning at 2–6 weeks.
• Baby is hungry, constipated and dehydrated. Loss of H^+ and Cl^- from stomach and K^+ from kidney causes hypochloraemic, hypokalaemic alkalosis.
• Palpable pyloric 'tumour' during a test feed or after vomiting.
• Gastric peristalsis may be seen. Ultrasound or Barium meal if diagnosis is uncertain.

Management
• Correct dehydration and electrolyte imbalance with 0.45% NaCl in dextrose 5% with added K^+. May take 24–48 hours to become normal.
• Ramstedt's pyloromyotomy via transverse RUQ or per umbilical incision. Normal feeding can commence within 24 hours.

Malrotation of the gut
Definition and aetiology
Malrotation describes a number of conditions that are caused by failure of the intestine to rotate into the correct anatomical position during embryological development. Midgut volvulus, internal herniae and duodenal and colonic obstruction may occur.

Clinical features
Bile-stained vomiting in the newborn period is the commonest presentation but older children may present with recurrent abdominal pain, abdominal distension and vomiting.

Management
Surgery is required to release the obstructions.

Meckel's diverticulum
Definition
Meckel's diverticulum is the remnant of the vitello-intestinal duct forming a blind-ending pouch on the antimesenteric border of the terminal ileum and is present in 2% of the population.

Clinical features
Most are asymptomatic. May present with rectal bleeding, mimic appendicitis (Meckel's diverticulitis), be a lead point for intussusception or cause a volvulus. Ectopic gastric mucosa in a Meckel's diverticulum is responsible for GI bleeding and may be detected by technetium pertechnate scan in 70% of cases.

Management
Surgical excision, even if found incidentally.

Intussusception
Definition
Intussusception is the invagination of one segment of bowel into an adjacent distal segment. The segment that invaginates is called the *intussusceptum* and the segment into which it invaginates the *intussuscepiens*. The tip of the intussusceptum is called the *apex* or *lead point*.

Aetiology
• 90% are idiopathic.
• Viral infection can lead to hyperplasia of Peyers patches which become the apex of an intussusception.

• Other lead points include Meckel's diverticulum, a polyp or a duplication cyst.

Clinical features
• Commonest cause of intestinal obstruction in infants 3–12 months. Males > females.
• Presents with pain (attacks of colicky pain every 15–20 min, lasting 2–3 min with screaming and drawing up of legs), pallor, vomiting and lethargy between attacks.
• Sausage-shaped mass in RUQ, empty RIF (sign de Dance).
• Passage of blood and mucus (redcurrant jelly stool).
• Tachycardia and dehydration.

Diagnosis
• Plain X-ray may show intestinal obstruction and sometimes the outline of the intussusception.
• Ultrasonography may help showing RUQ mass.
• Definite diagnosis by air or (less common) barium enema.

Management
• i.v. fluids to resuscitate infant (shock is frequent because of fluid sequesteration in the bowel).
• Air or barium reduction of intussusception if no peritonitis (75% of cases).
• Remainder require surgical reduction.

Inguinoscrotal conditions
Acute scrotum
Definition
The *acute scrotum* is a red, swollen, painful scrotum caused by torsion of the hydatid of Morgagni (60%), torsion of the testis (30%), epididimo-orchitis (10%) and idiopathic scrotal oedema (10%).

Management
• All cases of 'acute scrotum' should be explored.
• If true testicular torsion, treatment is bilateral orchidopexy (orchidectomy of affected testis if gangrenous).
• If torsion is hydatid of Morgagni, treatment is removal of hydatid on affected side only.

Inguinal hernia and hydrocele
Definition and aetiology
During the seventh month of gestation the testis descends from the posterior abdominal wall into the scrotum through a peritoneal diverticulum called the *processus vaginalis*, which obliterates just before birth.

An *inguinal hernia* in an infant is a swelling in the inguinal area due to failure of obliteration of the processus vaginalis, allowing bowel (rarely omentum) to descend within the hernial sac below the external inguinal ring.

A *hydrocele* is a collection of fluid around the testis that has trickled down from the peritoneal cavity via a narrow, but patent, processus vaginalis.

Diagnosis
• Diagnosis of a hydrocele is usually obvious: the scrotum contains fluid and transilluminates brilliantly.
• Diagnosis of a hernia may be entirely on the mother's given history or a lump may be obvious.
• Strangulation is a serious complication as it may compromise bowel and/or the blood supply to the testis.

Management
Both hernia and hydrocele should be treated by operation to obliterate the remaining processus vaginalis.

Undescended testis
Definition and aetiology
A *congenital undescended testis* (UDT) is one that has not reached the bottom of the scrotum at 3 months post-term. A *retractile testis* is one that can be manipulated to the bottom of the scrotum. An *ectopic testis* is one that has strayed from the normal path of descent.

Diagnosis
Most UDTs are found at the superficial inguinal pouch and associated with hypoplastic hemiscrotum and inguinal hernia.

Management
• Treatment is by orchidopexy and should be performed at 6–12 months.
• UDTs are at increased risk of developing malignancy, even after orchidopexy and require long-term surveillance.

Index

Page numbers in *italics* indicate figures; those in **bold** indicate tables.

ABC trauma sequence 78, 79
abdominal hernias 108–9
abdominal pain
  acute 28–9
  chronic 30–1
  referred 29
abdominal swellings 32–3
  generalized 33
  giant 32, 33
  lower 38–9
  upper 34–7
abdominal wall swellings 32, 33
achalasia 12, 13
acromegaly 128, 129
acute abdominal pain 28–9
acute renal failure 72–3, 77
Addisonian crisis 131
Addison's disease 130, 131
adhesions, intra-abdominal 30, 31
adrenal (suprarenal) gland
  disorders 130–1
  enlargement 35
  insufficiency 131
adrenogenital syndrome 131
airway obstruction 66, 67, 78, 79
amaurosis fugax 145
amputations 140
analgesia, postoperative 67
aneurysms 142–3
  aortic 37, 142, 143
  false (pseudo) 143
  femoral artery 48, 49
  subclavian artery 10, 11
  thrombosis 54, 55
angina pectoris 19, 134, 135
angiodysplasia 41
antibiotic-induced diarrhoea 45
antidiuretic hormone (ADH) deficiency 129
anuria 73
anus
  benign disorders 104–5
  bleeding 42, 43
  carcinoma 41
  discharge 104
  fissure 41, 105
  fistula 105
  lump 104
  see also perianal disorders
aortic aneurysms 37, 142, 143
  abdominal (AAA) 142, 143
aortic incompetence (regurgitation) 136, 137
aortic rupture 78
aortic stenosis 136, 137
aortoduodenal fistula 22, 23, 142
aorto-iliac occlusive disease 50, 51, 138
apnoea 67
appendicitis, acute 28, 96–7
appendix mass/abscess 38, 39, 96, 97

appendix testis, torsion 65
arterial disease, extracranial 144–5
arterial embolus 54, 55
arterial thrombosis 54, 55
arterial ulcers 56, 57
arteriovenous malformations, renal 63
ascites 32, 33
aspergilloma 14, 15
atelectasis 150–1
atheroma 51

Baker's cyst, ruptured 52, 53
Barrett's oesophagus 85
basal cell carcinoma (BCC), cutaneous 57, 132, 133
benign prostatic hypertrophy (BPH) 61, 63, 156–7
biliary colic 110, 111, 112, 113
bilirubin metabolism 40
bladder
  bleeding 62, 63
  masses 38, 39
  outflow obstruction 60, 61, 156
  stones 61, 63, 158, 159
  tumours (carcinoma) 58, 59, 61, 63, 162–3
blind loop syndrome (bacterial overgrowth) 45, 93
bone
  fractures 52, 53, 74–5
  tumours 52, 53
Bornholm's disease 18, 19
bowel habit, altered 46–7
  see also constipation; diarrhoea
brain injury
  primary 80, 81
  secondary 80, 81
branchial cyst 10, 11
breast
  abnormalities of normal development and involution (ANDI) 119
  abscess 17, 19, 119
  benign disease 118–19
  carcinoma 17, 21, 120–1
  cysts 17, 118, 119
  fat necrosis 17, 119
  fibroadenoma 16, 17, 119
  fibrocystic disease (FCD) 17, 19, 21, 118, 119
  lumps 16–17, 118
  pain 18–19
bronchial adenoma 14, 15
bronchial carcinoma 14, 15, 152–3
bronchiectasis 14, 15, 150
burns 76–7
  full thickness 76, 77
  partial thickness 76, 77
  Wallace's rule of 9's 76

caecum
  carcinoma 41, 42, 43, 102
  masses 39
calcium metabolism 126

cardiac failure 14, 15
cardiac tamponade 78
carotid artery disease 144, 145
carotid body tumour 10, 11
cauda equina lesion 51
caustic oesophageal stricture 12, 13
cellulitis 53
central nervous system (CNS) depression 66, 67
cervical lymphadenopathy 10, 11
cervical spine injury, potential 79
Chagas' disease 12, 13
chemical burns 77
children 170–1
cholangitis 110, 111, 112, 113
cholecystitis 110, 112
  acute 111, 113
  chronic 111, 113
cholera 45
Chvostek's sign 126, 127
cirrhosis of liver 35
Clarke's levels **133**
claudication
  intermittent 50–1, 139
  neurological 51
Clostridium difficile 45
coeliac disease 45, 93
colon
  bleeding 42, 43
  carcinoma 39, 43, 45, 47, 102–3
  masses 34, 36, 37, 38, 39
  polyps 43
colorectal carcinoma 102–3
compartment syndrome 74, 77
Conn's syndrome 131
constipation 46
  absolute 46
  acute 46
  chronic 33, 46, 47
contrecoup injury 80
coronary artery disease 135
cor pulmonale 150
costochondritis (Tietze's disease) 18, 19
Courvoisier's law 41, 117
cramps, muscle 53
Crohn's disease 45, 46, 93, 94–5
  inflammatory mass 39, 95
  perianal 43, 95
cryptorchidism (undescended testis) 48, 167, 171
Curling's ulcers 76, 77
Cushing's disease 129, 131
Cushing's syndrome 130, 131
cystic hygroma 10, 11
cystitis 154
  acute 58–9, 63
  interstitial 63
cystosarcoma phylloides 17

deep venous thrombosis (DVT) 53, 146–7
dermoid cysts 10, 11, 37

detrusor
  hyperreflexia 169
  instability *156*, *168*, 169
diabetes insipidus 129
diabetes mellitus *56*, 57, 61
diabetic foot 140–1
diarrhoea 44–5, 46
  spurious 45
Dieulafoy lesion *22*, 23
diverticular disease *42*, 43, 47, 98–9
diverticular mass *38*, 39
diverticulitis, acute 98, 99
Duke's staging system *102*
duodenal carcinoma, periampullary *116*, 117
duodenal ulcers 23, 25, *88*, 89
duodenitis 25
dysentery 45
dyspepsia 24–5
dysphagia 12–13
dysuria 58–9

ectopic pregnancy *38*, 39
electric burns 77
endocrine pancreatic tumours 117
enteritis 41
enuresis, nocturnal 169
epididymal cyst *64*, 65
epididymitis/epididymo-orchitis *64*, 65, 155
epidural analgesia 67
epiphyseal injuries *74*
escharotomy *76*, 77
extracranial arterial disease 144–5
extradural haemorrhage *80*, 82–3
eye, burns *76*, 77

faeces 33, 37, 39
fallopian tube, masses *38*, 39
fat
  malabsorption *92*, 93
  necrosis, breast 17, 119
femoral artery
  aneurysm *48*, 49
  stenosis *50*, 51
femoral hernia 48, 49, *108*, 109
femoral neuroma *48*, 49
femoro-popliteal arterial occlusion *50*, 51, *138*
fibroadenoma, breast *16*, 17, 119
fibrocystic disease (FCD), breast 17, 19, 21, *118*, 119
first aid 79
fissure *in ano* 41, 105
fistula *in ano* 105
flail chest 78
flank mass *160*
foot, diabetic 140–1
foreign body
  ingested *12*, 13
  inhaled *14*, 15
fractures *52*, 53, 74–5
  skull *80*, 82
frequency 45, 58
fungal nail infection *140*

galactocele 17
gallbladder
  empyema 35, *110*, *112*, 113
  enlargement *34*, 35
  mucocele 35, *110*, *112*

gallstone ileus 111
gallstones 25, 110–13
gastric carcinoma 23, 25, 37, 90–1
gastric ulcers 23, 25, *88*, 89
  Curling's *76*, 77
gastritis 23, 25
gastrointestinal (GI) bleeding 22, 42–3
gastro-oesophageal reflux 84–5
  in children 170
  disease (GORD) *12*, 13, 85
  see also oesophagitis, reflux
germ-cell tumours, testicular 167
giardiasis 45, *92*
Glasgow Coma Scale (GCS) 80, **81**, **83**
glomerulonephritis 63
gluten enteropathy (coeliac disease) 45, 93
goitre 122–3
gout 53
Graves' disease *122*, 123
Grawitz tumour (renal cell carcinoma) 35, 63, 160–1
groin swellings 48–9
gynaecomastia *118*, 119

haematemesis 22–3
haematuria 62–3, *160*
haemoglobinuria 63
haemoptysis 14–15
  spurious *14*, 15
haemorrhage *68*, 69, 79
  intracranial *80*, 81, 82–3
haemorrhoids 41, 104–5
haemothorax 78
head injury 80–3
heart disease
  ischaemic 134–5
  valvular 136–7
heart valves, prosthetic 137
Helicobacter pylori *88*, 89
hepatitis, infective 35
hereditary haemorrhagic telangiectasia *22*
hernias, abdominal 108–9
hiatus hernia 85
Hirschsprung's disease *46*, 47
hydatid cyst 35
hydatid of Morgagni, torsion *64*, 171
hydrocele *64*, 65, 171
  cordal 48
  femoral sac 49
hydronephrosis 35
hyperaldosteronism 131
hyperbilirubinaemia
  congenital 41
  conjugated *40*, 41
  unconjugated *40*, 41
hypercalcaemia *126*, 127
hypercalciuria 159
hypernephroma (renal cell carcinoma) 35, 63, 160–1
hyperparathyroidism *126*, 127
hyperprolactinaemia *128*
hyperthyroidism *122*, 123
hypocalcaemia *126*, 127
hypoparathyroidism 127
hypopituitarism 129
hypothyroidism *122*, 123
hypovolaemia *68*, 69, 73

hypoxaemia 67
hypoxia 66–7, *78*

iliac artery stenosis *50*, 51
incisional hernia 109
incontinence
  overflow 60, 169
  urinary 168–9
indigestion 25
infections
  in burned patients 77
  cervical lymphadenopathy 11
  leg *52*, 53, 57
  urinary tract (UTI) 58–9, 154–5
infective enterocolitis 44, 45, *46*
infra-popliteal occlusive disease *138*
inguinal hernia 65, *108*, 109
  direct 48, 109
  indirect 48, 109
  in infants 171
inguinal lymphadenopathy 48, 49
injuries *see* trauma
interleukins (IL-1α and IL-6) *70*, 71
intervertebral disc herniation 53
intestine
  lipodystrophy (Whipple's disease) *92*, 93
  malrotation 170
  obstruction 33, 106–7
  resection 93
  see also large bowel; small bowel
intracerebral haemorrhage *80*, 83
intracranial haemorrhage *80*, 81, 82–3
intracranial pressure, raised 27, *82*
intussusception 37, 41, 170–1
iodine deficiency 123
irritable bowel syndrome 30, 31, 45, *46*
ischaemia
  acute 54–5, 139
  chronic 51, *138*
  critical 139
  diabetic foot 141
ischaemic colitis *42*, 43
ischaemic enteropathy, chronic 93
ischaemic heart disease 134–5

jaundice 40–1
  haemolytic *40*, 41
  hepatic/hepatocellular *40*, 41
  obstructive *40*, 41, *110*, 111
joint trauma *52*, 53

kidney
  bleeding *62*, 63
  cysts 35, 63
  masses *34*, 35
  pelvic *38*, 39

lactorrhoea 21
Laplace's law 143
large bowel
  bleeding *42*, 43
  causes of diarrhoea 44, 45
  masses 36, 37, *38*, 39
  obstruction 27, 99, 107
  polyps *42*, 43, 45
laryngeal carcinoma *14*, 15
left atrial dilatation *12*

leg
  acute cold (ischaemia) 54–5
  acute warm painful 52–3
  postphlebitic (PPL) 146, 147
  referred pain 53
  trauma 52, 53, 54, 55
  ulceration 56–7, 140, 141
leiomyoma, stomach 22, 23
Leriche's syndrome 51
lipoma 17, 48
lipopolysaccharide (LPS) 70, 71
Lisfranc amputation 140
Littré's hernia 108
liver
  abscess 35
  enlargement 34, 35
lung
  abscess 14, 15, 150
  cancer see bronchial carcinoma
  empyema 150
  infarction 14, 15
  loss of functioning 66, 67
lymphadenopathy
  cervical 10, 11
  inguinal 48, 49
  mediastinal 12, 13
  retroperitoneal 36, 37

malabsorption 92–3, 95
Mallory–Weiss syndrome 22, 23
malrotation of gut 170
mammary duct
  ectasia 20, 21, 119
  papilloma 20, 21, 119
Marjolin's ulcer 57, 133
mastalgia 18, 19
mastitis 17, 19, 20, 21
Maydl's hernia 108
Meckel's diverticulum 31, 42, 170
mediastinal lymphadenopathy 12, 13
melaena 22
melanoma, malignant (MM) 57, 132, 133
mesenteric angina 31
micronutrient deficiencies 92
mitral incompetence (regurgitation) 136, 137
mitral stenosis 15, 136, 137
mouth, bleeding 15
multiple endocrine neoplasia (MEN)
  syndromes 125, 127
multiple organ dysfunction syndrome
  (MODS) 70, 71
muscle
  cramps 53
  trauma 53
myocardial infarction 134, 135

neck lumps 10, 11
nephroblastoma 35
neuropathic foot ulcers 56, 57, 141
nipple
  in breast cancer 120
  discharge 20, 21, 118
  Paget's disease 121
nitric oxide synthetase, inducible (iNOS) 71
nocturia 58
nocturnal enuresis 169
nose bleed 14, 15

obesity 33
oesophagitis, reflux 13, 23, 25, 84, 85
oesophagus
  Barrett's 85
  carcinoma 12, 13, 23, 25, 86–7
  pulsion diverticulum 13
  stricture 12, 13
  varices, bleeding 22, 23
oliguria 73
omentum, swellings 36, 37
opiate analgesia 67
oral tumours 14, 15
orchitis 64, 65
osteomyelitis 53, 140
ovary
  cysts 38, 39, 61
  masses 38, 39
overflow incontinence 60, 169

paediatric general surgery 170–1
Paget's disease of nipple 121
Pancoast's tumour 153
pancreas
  abscess 114, 115
  carcinoma 37, 116, 117
  endocrine tumours 117
  masses 34, 36, 37
  pseudocyst/cyst 37, 114, 115
  tumours 116–17
pancreatitis 111, 114–15
pan-hypopituitarism 129
paracolic abscess 39, 98
parasitic infections 93
parathormone 127
parathyroid gland
  disease 126–7
  localization 126
para-umbilical hernia 109
peau d'orange 121
pelvic masses 38, 39
peptic ulceration (PUD) 27, 88–9
  see also duodenal ulcers; gastric ulcers
periampullary carcinoma 116, 117
perianal disorders 104–5
  abscess 105
  in Crohn's disease 43, 95
  haematoma 105
  itch 104
  pain 47, 104
  see also anus
pericolic abscess 98
perinephric abscess 35
peripheral occlusive vascular disease 51, 57, 138–9
phaeochromocytoma 130, 131
piles (haemorrhoids) 41, 104–5
pilonidal sinus 105
pituitary gland
  disorders 128–9
  tumours 128, 129
platelet activating factor (PAF) 71
pleural effusion 150
pleurisy 18, 19
Plummer's disease 122
Plummer–Vinson syndrome 87
pneumaturia 58
pneumonia 14, 15, 28
  postoperative 150–1

pneumothorax, tension 78
polycystic kidney disease 35, 63
popliteal aneurysms 142, 143
postphlebitic limb (PPL) 146, 147
pregnancy 33, 38, 39, 47
  ectopic 38, 39
primary survey 79
processus vaginalis 171
proctitis 41, 101
prostate
  carcinoma 63, 164–5
  hypertrophy, benign (BPH) 61, 63, 156–7
prostatitis 155
pruritus ani (anal itch) 104
pseudomembranous colitis 45
psoas abscess 48, 49
pulmonary collapse 150–1
pulmonary embolus (PE) 146, 147
pulmonary hypertension 14, 150
pyelonephritis 58, 63, 154
pyloric stenosis 27, 89
  infantile hypertrophic 170
pyoderma gangrenosum 57
pyonephrosis 35
pyosalpinx 38

radiation
  burns 77
  enteropathy 93
Ranson's criteria 114
ray amputation 140
rectum
  bleeding 42–3, 104
  carcinoma 38, 39, 43, 102–3
  polyps 45, 46
  prolapse 105
  solitary ulcer 41
referred pain 29, 53
renal abscess 58, 154
renal calculi 63, 158–9
renal cell carcinoma (RCC) 35, 63, 160–1
renal colic 28, 159
renal failure, acute 72–3, 77
respiratory failure, neuromuscular 66
retching 26
retroperitoneal masses 35, 36, 37, 39
rheumatic fever 137
Richter's hernia 108
Riedel's lobe 35
road traffic accident (RTA) 79

salivary gland tumours 10, 11
Salmonella infections 45
salpingo-oophoritis 39
saphena varix 48, 49, 148
schistosomiasis 63
sciatica 53
scleroderma 12, 13
scrotum
  acute 171
  infantile oedema 65
  swellings 64–5
scurvy 15
sebaceous cyst 19, 65
secondary survey 79
seminoma 166, 167

sepsis 70
  syndrome 70
septic shock *68*, 69, 70
Sheehan's syndrome 129
Shigella infections 45
shock 68–9
  anaphylactic 69
  cardiogenic 69
  hypovolaemic *68*, 69
  septic *68*, 69, 70
Simmond's disease 129
skin cancer 57, 132–3
skull fracture *80*, 82
small bowel
  bacterial overgrowth (blind loop) 45, 93
  bleeding 42–3
  causes of diarrhoea *44*, 45
  ischaemia 41
  masses *36*, *38*, 39
  obstruction 27, 31, 107
  resection 93
  tumours 41
smoke inhalation *76*, 77
spermatic cord 48
spinal cord injuries 61
spleen, enlargement *34*, 35
squamous cell carcinoma (SCC), cutaneous 57,
  132, 133
staghorn calculi 159
sternocleidomastoid tumour *10*, 11
stomach
  distension 37
  hour-glass 27
  leiomyoma *22*, 23
  masses *34*, *36*, 37
  see also gastric carcinoma; gastric ulcers
stress incontinence *168*, 169
stroke 145
subclavian artery
  aneurysm *10*, 11
  ectasia *10*, 11
subclavian steal syndrome 145
subdural haemorrhage *80*, 83
suprarenal gland *see* adrenal (suprarenal)
  gland
Syme's amputation *140*
syphilis *64*, 65
systemic inflammatory response syndrome
  (SIRS) 70–1

telangiectasia, hereditary haemorrhagic
  22
teratoma, testicular *166*
testis
  ectopic 171
  haematocele 65
  retractile 171
  torsion *64*, 65, 171
  tumours *64*, 65, 166–7
  undescended (UDT, cryptorchidism) 48, 167,
    171
thrombosis *54*, 55
  aneurysm *54*, 55
  deep venous (DVT) 53, 146–7
  graft *54*, 55
thyroglossal cyst *10*, 11
thyroid gland
  benign hyperplasia 123
  malignancies 11, 124–5
  masses (swellings) *10*, 11
  solitary nodule 123, *124*
thyroiditis *122*, 123
Tietze's disease *18*, 19
torticollis 11
trachea
  bleeding *14*, 15
  carcinoma 12, *14*, 15
tracheo-oesophageal fistula *12*, 13
transient ischaemic attack (TIA) 145
transitional cell carcinoma (TCC) *38*, 39, 63,
  163
trauma
  head 80–3
  kidney 63
  leg 52, 53, *54*, 55, 57
  major (MT) 78–9
tricuspid regurgitation 137
tricuspid stenosis 137
Trousseau's sign *126*, 127
Trypanosoma cruzi (Chagas' disease) *12*,
  13
tuberculosis (TB)
  abdominal mass *38*, 39
  breast abscess 17, 21
  neck abscess *10*
  pulmonary *14*, 15
  renal 58, 63
  testis 65
tumour necrosis factor α (TNFα) 70, 71

ulcerative colitis 43, 45, 100–1
umbilical hernia 109
urachal cyst 39
ureter
  calculus 63, *158*, 159
  ectopic 169
ureteric (renal) colic *28*, 159
urethra
  calculus 61, 63
  obstruction *60*, 61
  trauma 63
urethral syndrome 59
urethritis 59
urge incontinence *168*, 169
urgency 45, 58
urinary calculi 63, 158–9
urinary fistula 169
urinary incontinence 168–9
urinary retention *38*, 39, 60–1
  acute 60
  chronic 60
  neurogenic 61
urinary tract infection (UTI) 58–9, 154–5
uterus
  carcinoma *38*, 39
  fibromyomas (fibroids) *38*, 39, 61
  masses *38*, 39

vaginitis 59
valvular heart disease 136–7
varicocele *64*, 65
varicose veins 148–9
vascular disease, peripheral occlusive 51, 57,
  138–9
vascular trauma 55, *74*
vasculitis *56*, 57
venous thrombosis, deep (DVT) 53, 146–7
venous ulcers *56*, 57, *148*
ventilation, poor *66*, 67
vertebrobasilar disease *144*, 145
vesicovaginal fistula *168*, 169
Virchow's triad *146*, 147
vitamin C deficiency 15
vitamin deficiencies *92*
vomiting 26–7

Wallace's rule of 9's *76*
waterbrash 26
Whipple's disease *92*, 93